OKANAGAN UNIV/COLLEGE LIBRARY

P9-EJI-954

850 .B85 1

PSYCHIATRIC DISORDERS ASSOCIATED WITH CHILDBIRTH

A GUIDE TO MANAGEMENT

ANNE BUIST

OKANAGAN UNIVERSITY COLLEGE
LIBRARY
BRITISH COLUMBIA

PSYCHIATRIC DISORDERS ASSOCIATED WITH CHILDBIRTH

A GUIDE TO MANAGEMENT

ANNE BUIST
MBBS, MMed, FRANZCP

McGRAW-HILL BOOK COMPANY Sydney
New York   San Francisco   Auckland   Bogotá
Caracas   Lisbon   London   Madrid   Mexico City
Milan   Montreal   New Delhi   San Juan
Singapore   Toronto

Notice
Medicine is an ever-changing science. As new research and clinical experience broaden our knowledge, changes in treatment and drug therapy are required. The editors and the publisher of this work have checked with sources believed to be reliable in their efforts to provide information that is complete and generally in accord with the standards accepted at the time of publication. However, in view of the possibility of human error or changes in medical sciences, neither the editor, nor the publisher, nor any other party who has been involved in the preparation or publication of this work warrants that the information contained herein is in every respect accurate or complete. Readers are encouraged to confirm the information contained herein with other sources. For example and in particular, readers are advised to check the product information sheet included in the package of each drug they plan to administer to be certain that the information contained in this book is accurate and that changes have not been made in the recommended dose or in the contraindications for administration. This recommendation is of particular importance in connection with new or infrequently used drugs.

Text © 1996 Anne Buist
Ilustrations and design © 1996 McGraw-Hill Book Company Australia Pty Limited

Apart from any fair dealing for the purposes of study, research, criticism or review, as permitted under the *Copyright Act*, no part may be reproduced by any process without written permission. Enquiries should be made to the publisher, marked for the attention of the Permissions Editor, at the address below.

Every effort has been made to trace and acknowledge copyright material. Should any infringement have occurred accidentally the authors and publishers tender their apologies.

Copying for educational purposes
Under the copying provisions of the *Copyright Act*, copies of parts of this book may be made by an educational institution. An agreement exists between the Copyright Agency Limited (CAL) and the relevant educational authority (Department of Education, university, TAFE, etc.) to pay a licence fee for such copying. It is not necessary to keep records of copying except where the relevant educational authority has undertaken to do so by arrangement with the Copyright Agency Limited.

For further information on the CAL licence agreements with educational institutions, contact the Copyright Agency Limited, Level 19, 157 Liverpool Street, Sydney NSW 2000. Where no such agreement exists, the copyright owner is entitled to claim payment in respect of any copies made.

Enquiries concerning copyright in McGraw-Hill publications should be directed to the Permissions Editor at the address below.

National Library of Australia Cataloguing-in-Publication data:

Buist, Anne Elizabeth
Psychiatric disorders associated with childbirth: a guide to management

Bibliography
Includes index
ISBN 0 07 470246 7.
1. Postpartum psychiatric disorders. 2. Postpartum psychiatric disorders—Treatment. 3. Mothers—Mental health. 4. Pregnancy—Psychological aspects. 5. Pregnant women—Mental health. I. Title.

618.76

Published in Australia by
McGraw-Hill Book Company Australia Pty Limited
4 Barcoo Street, Roseville NSW 2069, Australia
Sponsoring editor: John Rowe
Production editors: Karen Gray and Sarah Baker
Designer: Todd Pierce
Illustrator: Roy Bisson; cartoons based on ideas by R. Wade
Typeset in Australia by Craftsmen Type & Art
Printed in Australia by McPherson's Printing Group

Foreword

I have been treating women with postnatal psychiatric disorders for over 8 years. In that time there has been progress in the recognition of psychological disorders postpartum and of the short and long-term consequences, by both the public and health professionals. For a number of years, the Key Centre for Women's Health, University of Melbourne, has rotated all medical students through the Mercy Mother-Baby Unit, and has involved general practitioners in a training program in the managements of these disorders. There is still more to be done.

Many general practitioners, maternal-child health nurses, obstetricians and paediatricians are confronted by women with concurrent psychological symptoms during pregnancy and postpartum. This book is for them. With appropriate knowledge and awareness, many of these women can be managed in a primary care setting. Even when a psychiatrist is involved, appropriate management in the primary care setting is a crucial component of care. By improving our provision for this, we give women, their partners and their children a more optimistic outlook for the future.

Acknowledgments

Many thanks to my parents for their encouragement throughout my medical course, and to those who have supported me in putting together this book: my husband Graeme for tolerating the late nights of less than scintillating company, and our children, Daniel and Dominique, for sleeping! Special thanks for the review and suggestions by Klara Szego, Vickey Annakis, Leila Fazzalori and Francis Thomson-Salo; for the patience and dedication of Louise Ramsdell; and to my editors Bill Phippard and Susan Rintoul. Thanks also to all the staff members of the Mercy Hospital for Women Mother-Baby Unit for their unfailing professional and personal support.

About the author

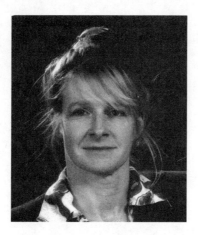

Dr Anne Buist is the Director of Psychological Medicine at the Mercy Hospital for Women and an Associate of the Key Centre for Women's Health, University of Melbourne. With Associate Professor Lorraine Dennerstein, she was responsible for the opening of the first mother-baby unit for postpartum psychological disorders in an obstetric hospital, at the Mercy.

Dr Buist is a prominent clinician and researcher in the area of postnatal psychiatric disorders. She was the first recipient of a Master of Medicine in Women's Health, at the University of Melbourne, looking at antidepressants and breastfeeding, and has just completed the first follow-up study of children exposed as infants to antidepressants through breast milk. She speaks frequently, Australia-wide and internationally, on postnatal depression and women's health issues.

Contents

CHAPTER 1

Postpartum psychiatric disorders: an overview

Introduction

Pregnancy and the postpartum period are often regarded as a time of joy, but this is not the experience for many women and their families.

The postpartum period is a time of great change for a woman. Throughout pregnancy her body has undergone alterations of function and shape, and the hormonal balance has shifted. These changes extend into the postpartum period with marked and sudden reduction in ovarian steroids, and breast enlargement and lactation in the breastfeeding woman. Menses may not return for some time. Emotionally there is also much upheaval, with changes in self-image, in the relationship with her partner, and in social circumstances which may involve moving from the paid and adult workforce to isolation at home. A further change occurs in moving from autonomy to accepting the dependence of a child.

Most women adapt to these changes, but it has been suggested that one or a combination of these changes is associated with a marked increase in the incidence of psychiatric illness in this period (Paffenberger 1964; Pitt 1968; Kendell et al 1976; Brandon 1982; Tonge 1984).

Psychiatric disorders specific to this period have been identified, although there is controversy about postpartum depression and psychosis, regarded by some as no different to depression and psychotic illnesses occurring at other times. Other clinicians and researchers in the area are concerned that many of these 'depressive illnesses' are related to the lack of societal support and the lowered status of motherhood, and abhor the overmedicalisation.

The postpartum or maternity blues is the most frequent presentation of emotional disturbance, affecting up to 80% of women. The transient and short-lived nature of the 'blues' means that there usually need be little intervention other than support and explanation (Hopkins et al 1984; Harding 1989).

Postpartum psychosis is in comparison relatively rare, occurring in 1–2 per 1000 births (Paffenberger 1964; Brockington et al 1981; Kendell 1985). Postpartum depression is quite common, however, with estimates from prospective studies of incidence generally between 10% and 20% (Paykel et al 1980; Cox et al 1982; Kumar & Robson 1984), but has been as high as 45% in an Australian sample (Tonge 1986).

Other psychiatric disorders also occur at this time. Although it is probably not more likely for these to occur for the first time in the postpartum period, women with a history of schizophrenia or manic depression will be at a higher risk of relapse due to stress, alterations in metabolism or dose of medication (for instance, lithium may have been stopped) and, possibly, hormonal changes. Eating disorders through pregnancy and postpartum present specific management issues for the obstetrician, paediatrician and psychiatrist.

There is a common theme in the management of these disorders. Unlike at any other life stage, particular consideration needs to be given to the woman and her partner's adjustment to parenthood, the relationship of the parents to the infant, the impact of biological treatments on the infant in utero and whether the infant is breastfed. The impact of the illness on the family should be considered at all times in the management of psychiatric disorder. This is particularly crucial in the first few years of a child's life.

Postpartum blues

Postpartum, maternity or baby blues is generally accepted as a common accompaniment to childbirth. The incidence has been estimated at between 50% and 80% (Yalom et al 1968; Pitt 1973; Hopkins et al 1984; Tonge 1986; Condon & Watson 1987). The syndrome is characterised by lowered mood, anxiety, tearfulness, irritability, insomnia and fatigue. It usually begins 3 to 5 days postpartum and lasts for from hours to days at most (Pitt 1973; Harding 1989; Steiner 1990). These symptoms are reported to have varying significance and there is little consensus regarding this (Kennerley & Gath 1986).

It has been suggested that there may be a link between postpartum blues and the development of subsequent postpartum depression, with a possible similar aetiological bond (Kendell et al 1981; Hapgood et al 1988). Hapgood's study found that women with severe lability of mood were at the highest risk, and that this lability appeared unpredictable by demographic data. This study may have been identifying a particular subgroup prone to postpartum depression. Some other studies have failed to replicate this relationship (Kumar & Robson 1984), but an international prospective collaborative study has also found a strong relationship between the occurrence of postpartum blues and later postpartum depression (Dennerstein et al 1989).

Postpartum psychosis

Postpartum psychosis is the most severe and least common of the puerperal disorders. It has been referred to by Hippocrates, and described in detail by

Esquirol and Marce in the 19th century. Its incidence is estimated at 1–2 per 1000 births (Paffenberger 1964; Brockington 1981; Kendell 1985). The onset is generally abrupt, and commonly within the first month postpartum, particularly the first week (Paffenberger 1964; Protheroe 1969; Brockington et al 1981).

The definition of this disorder is unclear. Described symptoms include hallucinations, delusions, disorganisation (Harding 1989), clouding of consciousness (Protheroe 1969; Brockington et al 1981) and manic-depressive mood swings (Brockington et al 1981). There is particular confusion because of varying opinions on whether or not it is a distinct entity.

Reports have tended to categorise the illness as either schizophrenia or major affective disorder. Early work in the area implied that postpartum psychosis was a form of schizophrenia (Bleuler 1911; Kraeplin 1913); however, later research supports the current view that most of these presentations are affective in type.

Protheroe (1969) described 134 cases, of which he categorised 91 as affective reactions, 37 as schizophrenia and 6 as organic. Brockington et al (1981), using research diagnostic criteria, reported 58 cases occurring in the first month postpartum, of which 14 were diagnosed with schizophrenia, 16 as schizo affective, 18 manic, 7 mixed affective and 3 undiagnosed.

Brockington et al (1981) described postpartum psychosis as usually being florid affective episodes, with hallucinations, marked emotional lability and significant manic symptoms.

Other researchers agree that schizophrenia is relatively rare among the postpartum psychoses—between 2% and 16% (Dean & Kendell 1981; Meltzer & Kumar 1985).

The association with affective illness is also seen in studies evaluating risk factors. A history of psychosis, either puerperal or non-puerperal, is viewed as a major risk factor, and this is particularly so if the psychosis was affective (Kendell 1985; Kendell et al 1987; Reich & Winokur 1970). There is also an increased incidence of a family history of affective psychotic illness (Paffenberger 1982; O'Hara 1987).

A majority of opinion appears to be that puerperal psychosis is an affective variant (Brockington & Cox-Roper 1982; Steiner 1990) with a better prognosis than non-puerperal psychosis, fewer relapses and fewer suicides (Platz & Kendell 1988). Dean and Kendell (1981) compared puerperal and non-puerperal psychosis and found the former group to be more disoriented, more labile and more agitated.

Nosological systems currently do not give consideration to postpartum psychosis being in any way different from psychosis occurring at other times. Early systems made some allowance. The International Classification of Diseases (ICD 8) included 'unspecified psychosis occurring within six weeks of delivery' but this was no longer present in the ICD 9, or the Diagnostic and Statistical Manual of Mental Disorder (DSM IIIR) (Brockington & Cox-Roper 1982). The lack of agreement on specific criteria has created considerable difficulties in research. Comparison of studies using different diagnostic criteria is difficult. Clinically, patients may not fit well into current categories, and prognosis and outcome may be quite different.

Postpartum depression

The nosological difficulties with postpartum psychosis are manifested to an even greater degree with postpartum depression. It is often included with postpartum psychosis, confused with the 'blues' and is not included in either the International Classification of Diseases (ICD 10, 1992) or the Diagnostic and Statistical Manual of Mental Disorder (DSM IV, 1994).

Using the latter's criteria for depression, postpartum depression may be classified as a major depression, atypical depression, adjustment disorder or even dysthymia. Amid this confusion, researchers use a variety of diagnostic criteria when evaluating the disorder, at times contributing to conflicting results (Steiner 1990).

Incidence

Largely because of the difficulties in definition, estimates of incidence of postpartum depression vary, with the most commonly accepted figure at 10–15% (Kumar & Robson 1984; O'Hara et al 1984; Cox et al 1982).

Timing of interviews, and depression criteria appear crucial; self-report is associated with higher reported incidences. This is highlighted in Dennerstein et al's study (1989) where, on self-report, 43% of women noted depression in the previous 4 months. With the Beck Depression Inventory, assessment at this time, however, demonstrated an incidence of 14%.

Arguments about whether postpartum depression is a discrete entity have focused on whether the incidence is any different among postpartum women when compared to non-puerperal controls. Cooper et al (1988) concluded prevalence rates to be the same. Other studies have found differences (Cox et al 1982; Kumar & Robson 1984).

Onset

The onset of symptoms is generally reported at before 4 to 6 weeks (O'Hara et al 1984; Kumar & Robson 1984; Tonge 1984; Steiner 1990). In Tonge's 1984 study women were 6 times more likely to become depressed in the first 4 weeks than in subsequent months. However, presentation is frequently later, even after another pregnancy and further deterioration, or not at all. The delayed presentation may reflect a number of factors: the illness may often be missed or misdiagnosed due to confusion with 'blues', and a belief that depression at this time is a sociopolitical problem of changing roles. The women themselves frequently cover up symptoms, being at a loss to understand their feelings.

Clinical features

Controversy exists over whether symptoms of postpartum depression differ from those of other major depressive illnesses. Mood disturbance may or may not be a major presenting symptom (Oppenheim 1983), but tearfulness, irritability, feelings of inadequacy, poor concentration and inability to cope with even minor tasks are common. Guilt and anxiety are frequently reported, along with feelings of failure as a mother. The baby may be the focus of anxiety or of obsessional thoughts of harm, which adds further to the, at times, overwhelming guilt. Decreased libido, exhaustion and appetite disturbance are also reported. Sleep disturbance may become manifest as difficulty getting to sleep, and early morning wakening (Oppenheim 1983; Cox 1983; Pauleikhoff 1987).

Duration and outcome

O'Hara and Zekoski (1988) report a duration of 1 to 6 weeks, but other investigators have found women to be depressed throughout the first year postpartum (Pitt 1968; Kumar & Robson 1984; Cox et al 1982). Depression has been reported to be longstanding with on-going difficulties for up to 4 years (Uddenberg & Englesson 1978; Wolkind et al 1980; Kumar & Robson 1984).

The protracted course of some of these depressions has potentially devastating effects on the woman, her partner and her child, and emphasises the need for rapid diagnosis and appropriate management (Uddenberg & Englesson 1978; Puckering 1989; Steiner 1990). In other studies some correlation has been found between maternal depression and the child's poorer cognitive performance (Coghill et al 1986), behavioural disturbances and negative mother–child interaction (Caplan et al 1989). Coghill et al's study (1986) and others (Richman et al 1982; Mills & Meadows 1987) have highlighted that it is earlier depression, not current depression, that appears important. They suggest that early impairment of the mother–child relationship sets a course that is not easy to alter. Some studies have not found a relationship between maternal depression and impairment of the child's development (Wrate et al 1985; Ghodsian et al 1984), but the concern generated from the more recent studies has led to considerable interest and current research.

Aetiology

A number of aetiological theories of postpartum blues/depression/psychosis have been postulated. There remains no consensus as to the cause, and it seems likely to be multifactorial. Methodological difficulties and the complexity of the postpartum period from each of the biological, psychological and social aspects appear to be major factors in establishing the relative contributions of these factors to the aetiology. These will be discussed more fully in subsequent chapters.

CHAPTER 2

Basic counselling skills

Introduction

Counselling and therapy in various forms are done all the time by many health professionals—although they don't always know that they are doing it! Being a 'therapist' has achieved a certain mystique. To do a specific 'pure' therapy such as psychoanalysis or cognitive behavioural therapy, study and supervision over years is required. Therapy of an analytic/psychodynamic nature should be left to specialists, who deal with people with (usually) a very troubled past.

Many women with anxiety and depressive disorders through pregnancy and the postpartum—and their families—can benefit from a simpler and basic counselling which can be supplied by a variety of health professionals, providing they have:

1. the interest;
2. the ability to establish a therapeutic relationship;
3. the time—for, on occasion, long and frequent appointments;
4. an overall understanding of the condition;
5. the availability of a specialist for secondary liaison or assessment;
6. sound clinical judgment—knowing when to involve a specialist.

The background

1. The relationship, crucial to counselling, starts from before the first interview; before the woman sees you, she has ideas about what your role and capacity is. This can work positively—or negatively. It may be related to your job title (for instance, doctor, maternal-child health nurse) and/or your gender. It may also be affected by previous experiences with someone from your professional group.

   Many of these women are feeling anxious and are lacking self-esteem. They feel easily intimidated and, if their husband is not supportive and the therapist is male, may presume that the therapist will also be unable to understand how they feel.

2. The therapist also brings with them preconceived ideas which may affect what is asked and what is heard. Beware of gender or race stereotypes. Be aware of your own posture, facial expressions and your feelings, particularly of empathy and understanding.

   Practical points, such as sitting to the side of your desk rather than having it separate you from the woman, can help promote a closer therapeutic relationship. Interruptions by other staff or by telephones ringing should be avoided where possible. The woman needs to feel that you want to listen and that she has, briefly, your undivided, emphatic attention.

3. At the first interview:
   - introduce yourself;
   - ask open-ended questions;
   - allow the woman plenty of time to respond;
   - if she is presenting her child as the problem, don't forget to inquire gently how the woman is feeling;
   - listen to her words (are they consistent with how she appears, how she is acting and responding?);
   - if you feel there is more than is being said, ask gently if there is anything else, but do not push;
   - let her know your future availability.

4. The frequency of appointments will depend on severity, and may fluctuate. Accommodate this as well as possible. If you are going on leave, be sure to let the woman know well ahead of time and, where possible, introduce her to your relief.

5. Be aware of your own feelings towards the woman. These may change over time, and include despair, anger and frustration. Ask yourself if these are 'your' feelings, or is it something that the woman is 'projecting' on to you? It is very easy to feel the situation is hopeless, when the woman is relaying long horrific life details where she feels she is the victim; as the health professional it is important to acknowledge these feelings, and feel what it must be like for her, but also to rise above this, to be objective.

Basic skills

Educative

Women and their families generally have little—or an incorrect—knowledge about psychological disorders. Even if they have been provided with pamphlets, and identify themselves with the listed symptoms, there are still many unanswered questions about aetiology, management, course and prognosis. Be sure to do the following:

1. Make the diagnosis.
2. Outline the likely causes (usually multifactorial). Be optimistic (but truthful) about the prognosis. Discuss management options.
3. Encourage questions at first, and subsequent visits.

4. Where possible, let the woman and her family make decisions about management. Women with psychological disorders may have difficulty making decisions, so may have to be guided by what is *generally* done and what is *usually* helpful.

5. Reinforce the notion that there are things that the woman herself can do to help herself get better. 'Medicalisation' of a disorder, and the old-fashioned view of the doctor knowing best and handing out the medicine bottle, may temporarily bring relief, but promotes the feeling of powerlessness and helplessness, which may reinforce a low self-esteem in these women.

6. Empower the woman—help her to take responsibility for her symptoms, her treatment and her recovery.

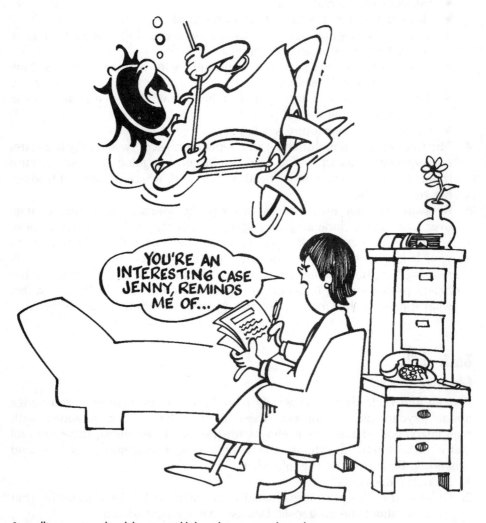

Counselling requires the ability to establish a therapeutic relationship

Support

1. Unconditional, uncritical support is something many people do not have; it is particularly important for a woman with psychological disorders at this very vulnerable life phase to feel she has this from someone. Where her partnership is strained, or where the woman has issues, particularly from her childhood, that she does not wish to share with her partner (often due to guilt or shame), a health professional is in a good position to provide this. 'Unconditional' and 'uncritical' does *not* mean that any type of behaviour is condoned but rather that there is an acceptance of the goodness and worth of the person, and an understanding of other aspects.

2. Support may require long or frequent interviews, but it must be realistic. Don't offer something you are unable to deliver. Remember that you can promise to help them, but it is not in your power to 'cure' them.

3. In a supportive role, it can be important to just be a 'sounding' board at times. Sometimes women do not expect an immediate or practical solution. Just feeling someone has listened to and understood them can be therapeutic. You may also be providing a role model (mother/father) for them which they lack in their own family.

4. While giving dogmatic advice is not helpful, offering suggestions can be. As a health professional you have the advantage of looking at the situation from the outside, and can offer quite a different perspective on the situation. You are not limited by the disorder, or the family and psychological pressures to which the woman is exposed; it may be possible to reframe situations from a different perspective, and suggest solutions which the woman has not considered.

   For instance, a distressed, depressed woman who banishes her 3-year-old to his room for bad behaviour finds he has wet his bed. This is regarded as an act of defiance by the child, and further angers the mother. This could be reframed as an act of fear—and the child's loss of control (urinary) mirroring his mother's loss of (emotional) control. Rather than increased punishments, increased positive attention reinforcing the mother being in control may resolve the on-going problems.

Family intervention

As the health professional, you see the woman for very small periods of time compared to her family. Family members are important sources of information, and can be important as supports. To be supportive, they need to understand the situation, and how they can help. This information is better supplied by a health professional than by the woman herself. Be aware that the family dynamics can negatively affect the course of the illness; if this appears to be the case, refer to a family therapist.

Cognitive techniques

To effectively undertake cognitive behavioural therapy, study, training and supervision is required; however, many basic techniques can be helpful in

the day-to-day management of the depressive and anxiety disorders that are common in the postpartum. They are not of value in the management of psychosis. With the direction of the therapist, these techniques help the woman to identify the cognitions (thoughts) that precipitate/are associated with her symptoms, and any resulting maladaptive behaviours. People who are depressed/anxious characteristically have thoughts which:
- are predominantly negative, focusing on the bad rather than the good (for instance, the half-empty tank rather than the half-full);
- are overgeneralised (for instance, *I always mess things up*);
- are catastrophic;
- lack perspective.

While there is controversy about whether such thinking causes depression, or vice versa, helping women to identify these thought processes helps them to understand their feelings, and empowers them. There is good evidence that it also helps them to get better.

Any 'cognitive' techniques will need to be reinforced regularly. Self-help books (for instance, I. Marks (1980) *Living with Fear.* US: McGraw-Hill, or A. Ellis and R. Harper (1975). *A New Guide to Rational Living.* Wiltshire Book Company with Prentice-Hall) consulted daily if possible, can also benefit women.

Here are some useful techniques:
1. Help the woman identify the thoughts that are worrying her. For instance, a woman reports that every time her child cries, she becomes increasingly agitated.
    - What is it about the child's cry that evokes this response?
    - What does the cry mean to her?
    - She tells you that she is afraid she will be unable to settle the infant, or that she won't know what is wrong with it.
    - Does it really matter if she doesn't?

    She may fear that she might lose control and harm the child. Or that by being unable to settle the child, by not 'knowing instinctively' what is wrong, that this means she is a bad mother—as she is if she does harm, or even thinks of harming, her child (or wishes it had never been born).

    The thoughts that are preoccupying this woman are that she is a bad mother, that she has 'failed'.

    A diary may be helpful. Get the woman to note the times when she feels worst. Ask her to note what has happened and what she is thinking.
2. Help the woman challenge her negative/illogical thoughts: for instance, do mothers always know what is wrong with their babies?
    - Did her mother know? Did her mother-in-law? Her next-door neighbour? Do her friends know? *Always?*
    - If her friend couldn't settle her child, would that make *her* a bad mother?
    - If there are repetitive themes, get the woman to write down 3 or 4 logical responses and to look at these *every time* she experiences those negative thoughts.

3. Help the woman identify the expectations she has of herself. Are they realistic? For instance, a mother of 3 expects to have her floors and ovens cleaned every day, as well as doing the regular housework, making nutritious meals, shopping, transporting children to school and/or kindergarten, regularly entertaining 10 or more of her husband's clients and doing her father's ironing. When she is unable to do so, she feels she has failed.
   - Ask her if she knows anyone who does this?
   - Point out that if she is exhausted, she may be unable to spend good 'quality' time with her children.
   - Ask her to make a list of priorities.
   - Ask her to expect to get only 3 or 4 of the most important tasks completed—and to congratulate herself on any extra tasks achieved.

4. Reinforce perspective; saying that 'things could be worse' is not always well received, but is almost always true. Depressed/anxious people are trapped in their own world by their own fears; sometimes it is the fear of something happening rather than the reality with which they are unable to deal. Hypochondriacs, terrified for years by the thought of illness, can often cope quite well when a real medical illness is diagnosed. Help the woman challenge whether what she fears will ever happen and, even if it does, will it be that bad?

   For instance, a woman states that she fears that if her child cries continuously, she might harm it.
   - Has she ever?
   - If not, what has stopped her?
   - Are there things (for instance, walking away and leaving the child in its cot until she is feeling calmer) she can do to prevent this?
   - If she did 'harm' her child what does she think she would have done, realistically?

   Often these depressed/anxious women are obsessional and rigidly in control. They may be, in fact, certain that they wouldn't harm the child, but feel guilty that the thought has ever crossed their mind. (If you are concerned that they actually might harm the child, refer for admission/ urgent specialist assessment.) 'Harm' may mean a lot of things of varying severity and, if pressed, the worst that they think would *actually* happen might be yelling in frustration.

5. Humour can be a worthwhile tool if used appropriately by the therapist. It can also be encouraged in the women—it helps decrease tension, and reinforces a sense of perspective. So—the car broke down, you lost your job, and the cat got run over. Yes, it could have been better—your car could have been stolen (and you could have claimed on its insurance), it could have been your ex-boss who got run over and your cat could have got the flu—but hell, you needed a new job, why not sell the car, you never liked it, and at least you don't have to worry about a vet's bill. There are more important things—your health, your family's health and so on.

Anxiety management

Anxiety is a common feature of postnatal depression (PND). It may present in a number of ways: physical symptoms such as excessive perspiration, hyperventilation, shaking, muscle tension, nausea, diarrhoea and headaches, or with fears usually associated with self or infant. These may include a fear of not coping, of going mad or of harming the infant, or a fear for the infant's health. The level of anxiety can fluctuate, and may have identifiable precipitants. These may be associated with panic attacks, that is, specific episodes, usually brief, of intense physical and psychological symptoms of anxiety.

1. Anxiety can be debilitating, and difficult to treat; it is important to take the symptoms seriously, and to let the woman know she can get over these feelings and that help is available.

2. If symptoms are severe, and particularly if they are associated with a depression or panic disorder, medication may be appropriate. Where possible, avoid minor tranquillisers. Antidepressant medication can have some anti-anxiety effects and it is preferable to minimise the number of medications used. A sedative tricyclic can give immediate benefit, but the sedation for some is intolerable; other antidepressants can address the anxiety but it may take some weeks to see the benefit. Knowing that things will improve, plus basic anxiety management techniques, can help the woman through these weeks. As an alternative, low doses of short-term anxiolytics can be considered. The exception here is a woman with a clear panic disorder, where referral to a psychiatrist should be made.

3. Help the woman to identify what precipitates the anxiety, what it is that she actually fears, by going through the thought processes one at a time. Avoiding the precipitant (if there is one identifiable), while it might avoid a major panic attack, may worsen the situation overall. In some situations the woman can be helped to challenge her fear—that 'the worst that could happen' is perhaps not as bad as she thinks. And that the worst is not going to happen. Many of the thoughts underlying anxiety are illogical—they need to be continually challenged by logic and a sense of perspective (see cognitive techniques on pp. 9–11).

4. Ask the woman if there is anything she does which relieves the anxiety, such as taking a walk, or having a shower. Help the woman plan what she will do next time she gets anxious. It is often difficult to go for a walk at certain times, but standing in the back garden may help. If the precipitant of the anxiety is a crying baby who has failed to settle, it is preferable that the woman leave the infant (safely in a cot) and distance herself briefly, than leave herself exposed to a situation with which she is unable to deal, where she may harm (or feel like harming) the infant. Ten minutes out of earshot of the infant, having a cup of coffee, taking deep breaths and reassessing the situation will help the woman feel she is remaining in control.

5. Relaxation tapes are commercially available; relaxing music is an alternative. These tapes can be used in times of crisis, but should also be

used on a daily, regular basis. The greater the anxiety, the harder it is to benefit from the tapes—having the woman bring her own tape, and making a specific tape for her, while she relaxes on the consulting room couch, can increase its effectiveness. These tapes do not need to be long (10 to 20 minutes is sufficient), and the voice needs to be quiet and steady. Visual imagery or gradual relaxation of each body part can be used. If visual imagery is used, it is important to discuss this with the woman first—ask her what scene or place she would find relaxing (for instance, a beach, or forest). Such a scene is then described on the tape, with the woman described as feeling relaxed, having no worries and being in control. At the end of the tape, it is important to say that the woman will awake and feel completely alert. A small percentage of the population is highly susceptible to hypnosis and may 'self-hypnotise' in such situations. Such people may take a little longer to return to a fully alert state, and should remain in the office until they have done so.

6. Failure to improve: while many women with milder disorders will respond to these basic techniques, others will not. Where there is failure to improve or the situation is deteriorating:
   - reassess the diagnosis;
   - consider what psychosocial factors may be perpetuating the illness (for instance, is there any secondary gain?);
   - refer to a psychiatrist/psychologist, preferably one with experience in the management of psychological disorders in pregnancy and the postpartum.

CHAPTER 3

Becoming a parent

Becoming pregnant

The transition to parenthood begins long before the arrival of a child. In Western society, contraception allows most women a degree of choice. The choice, however, may not be straightforward, rather a mixture of conscious or unconscious desires and fears. Unplanned pregnancies still occur, and while the option of termination may be available and adopted, other women continue with the pregnancy, sometimes reluctantly. Increased societal acceptance of and government support for single mothers has resulted in a marked increase in women keeping babies who would have been adopted in previous eras; this has relieved the burden of guilt but brought on-going responsibility—for some, overwhelming responsibility.

Unplanned pregnancy and negative attitudes to motherhood have been linked to depression in some studies (Condon & Watson 1987). Kumar and Robson (1984) linked severe doubts about having the baby to both antenatal and postnatal depression but concluded that the women tended to have depression either antenatally or postnatally but not both. The pregnancy may awaken feelings from childhood, the woman's relationship to her own parents, her self-concept and future aspirations. Some, who choose termination, may leave these issues aroused but unresolved, to declare themselves in subsequent pregnancies.

Women who choose to become pregnant and to continue a pregnancy may do so for many reasons. Societal or spouse pressure, relief from the tedium of a job, the biological clock and fears of being unable to reproduce, necessitating an urgency, may be important. Brazelton and Cramer (1991) identify common psychological needs associated with pregnancy: identification with one's own mother and need to replace and to separate from her; the wish to be 'complete'; mirroring oneself in the child and expecting the child to fulfil one's own lost ideals and opportunities. The degree of importance of these reasons varies between women; establishing what these fantasies are may be important in women who present through pregnancy and the postpartum with a variety of physical and emotional difficulties. In taking a history, remember to ask if the pregnancy was planned, and how well the woman feels she and her partner accepted the pregnancy. Most women will say that by later in the pregnancy they had come to terms with, and wanted, the child. Earlier ambivalence may re-emerge in the stress of the postpartum period.

Case example

Donna, 25, had been married for 5 years. She worked as a legal clerk, and found her job repetitive and unstimulating, but felt that she was unqualified and was too unsure of herself to leave. Her husband, Stan, worked long hours in his own video shop. He was from a traditional Greek background, and felt she should 'stay at home and have children'. Donna was an only child, and her parents quietly pressured her for grandchildren.

Donna was admitted twice in early pregnancy with hyperemesis, and was referred for psychiatric opinion; the obstetrician felt that there were marital problems.

Donna described having been off contraception for over a year, but appeared ambivalent about the notion of pregnancy and was excessively fearful of childbirth. She had had to leave work because of severe nausea and vomiting and had moved in with her mother temporarily because 'Stan was never at home'.

At subsequent interviews, Donna appeared increasingly anxious, and very defensive of her husband. She spoke of wanting a girl 'just like me' who would 'do things differently'. When asked what she meant by this, she was initially evasive, then broke down in tears, confessing that she was unsure who the child's father was. Three months prior to becoming pregnant, she had begun an affair with a married friend of her husband's—in part in frustration at not becoming pregnant as she had expected, but more to express her anger at her husband for neglecting her. The result—a child—had major ramifications for Donna's mental health, and her capacity to relate to the child. Her ability to continue in an unsatisfactory relationship was further compromised. Her refusal to have on-going psychiatric help represented an attempt at denial that is unlikely to be wholly, if at all, successful.

The pregnancy

The incidence of psychiatric illness decreases during the period of pregnancy itself (Kendell et al 1987). The woman is required to deal with marked physiological changes; the initial euphoria may be quickly deflated by 'morning sickness', fatigue and weight gain. For women with body-image disturbances, such as those with a history of anorexia or bulimia nervosa, this weight gain may represent a very real stress. Repeated patterns of inadequate food intake, self-induced vomiting and laxative abuse will carry significant risks to the foetus; others will respond with tense, carefully monitored minimum weight gains, so that the baby's health is less likely than the mother's to be affected. Careful obstetric care is essential, and vitamin supplements are an important consideration.

The woman and her partner must also come to terms with the reality of becoming parents. Idealisation of the baby, and of themselves as parents, is common. Hormonal influences direct the woman to become more introspective: the Primary Maternal Preoccupation of which Winnicott (1956) speaks assists in attachment to the infant. With foetal movements, the baby becomes very real and the mother may identify strongly with the infant. It is common for women to worry about the health of their infant, about childbirth and about the future. Excessive anxiety has been associated with the later development of depression in some studies (Cutrona 1982; Dennerstein et al 1989) and may represent the beginnings of psychological maladjustment in coming to terms with being a mother.

Women with a history of psychotic disorder are at risk of deterioration as a result of the stress of pregnancy or cessation of medication (discussed in Chapter 8). Women with bipolar disorder are at particular risk because of the cessation of lithium. Women with schizophrenia are prone to relapse; delusional ideas may relate to their changed bodily sensations, and it is common for them to be ambivalent towards the child (Spielvogel & Wile 1986; McNeil et al 1984). These women are also more likely to be noncompliant with antenatal care, including being at risk of self-neglect and poor diet, with potential ramifications for the child. These women and their pregnancies should be carefully monitored where possible—easier in an in-patient setting, but otherwise with the co-operation of a member of the family or a visiting psychiatric team taking women to antenatal appointments.

Fathers-to-be

Like his pregnant partner, becoming a parent presents a challenge to the man, the resolution of which will be affected by his own background, the relationship with his partner and the significance of the pregnancy. Pregnancy may be reassuring in terms of the man's potency, and brings fantasies of a child (usually a son) who will reinforce his own self-image. It may also be frightening: tightening a net about an ambivalent commitment, increasing a sense of responsibility and severing ties to a carefree youth.

Unlike the woman, the man is not constantly reminded of the pregnancy. He only feels the child when his partner's hand guides him; and he does not have the hormonal influence centring him on the child. For some men, physical symptoms are experienced; some 14% suffer from some form of couvade syndrome (Trethowan & Conlon 1965), which consists of lowered appetite, nausea or vomiting, headache or toothache. It is thought that this may represent identification with, or ambivalent feelings to, the man's partner and child.

Most commonly, the father-to-be will experience a sense of exclusion (Brazelton & Cramer 1991). The focus of attention is on the woman—and hers is on the infant. This accentuates towards term, and worsens post-delivery. Although the trend of antenatal classes is now to include the fathers, and in Western culture they are now expected to be at the birth, this can be overwhelming and unwelcomed by some men, recent research suggests (Barclay 1994).

Men react differently to the changes in their partners. Those in a supportive and intimate relationship may be able to remain in tune with their partners, and continue to develop their relationship. A relationship such as this is strongly predictive of a smoother transition to parenthood and less risk of postpartum depression (Grossman et al 1980). Brown (1986) looked at marital support in pregnancy, and found interest in and sharing of the pregnancy, reassurance of needs and the provision of support were generally well met; men, however, felt that their partners were not understanding of the difficulties that changes in the sexual relationship entailed. This is a theme that can continue into the postpartum, and heightens the feelings of exclusion in the male; the sexual relationship often becomes less of a focus for the woman, whose physical and emotional needs are being largely met by the pregnancy and foetus and then the infant, and probably breastfeeding. Through pregnancy the man is expected to understand this—in the postpartum it is often left to him to persuade his partner of the importance of their own intimate relationship. This requires maturity in both the new parents. Where the relationship is strained, or where one or both partners is unable or unwilling to tackle the tasks required, some men may react by having affairs, or by separating themselves with alcohol, sport or work. Sensible pregnancy planning, or sensitive intervention in pregnancy, acknowledging the importance and difficulties of the father's role (rather than adding to the expectations as in current antenatal classes) may help avert many later difficulties, although such work may need to continue into the postpartum when the stress of the reality itself eventuates.

Case example

Rita, 36, and Jon, 32, married after knowing each other for 6 months. A year after their marriage, Rita became pregnant. She described a sense of panic induced by seeing all her other friends having children, but admitted that she had never been a maternal person; when she found out that she was pregnant she cried. Jon was quiet and comforting—and left her 3 months later. Rita had 'no idea' why.

A month prior to the birth, Rita and Jon were reconciled. Although well through the pregnancy, Rita developed a severe depression in the first week postpartum.

When Rita presented, she described feeling that she had made a mistake and felt hopeless and helpless regarding the future. She appeared unmotivated to get better, clearly feeling that Jon had returned to her through a sense of guilt, and now remained only to support her through her illness.

Jon was reluctant to be involved in therapy. He conveyed a sense of being uncommitted to the relationship—but was caring of his son. He spoke of a feeling of dread that had descended on him when Rita had said that she was pregnant; her tears had been reminiscent of those of his own mother, who had been depressed throughout his childhood. He described his father as aloof and authoritarian and said that his mother had relied on him, Jon, emotionally. To Jon, becoming a father was a re-creation of his own childhood, from which he still felt he needed to escape. The short time he and Rita had had together before the pregnancy had been inadequate to establish any firm and intimate link—and ultimately, after Rita's illness improved, they separated. The issues arising from becoming a father made Jon aware of many repressed feelings with which he knew he needed to deal before considering becoming a father again.

Special pregnancies

The decision to have a baby does not always result in either pregnancy or a live, healthy child. With markedly improved obstetric intervention this century, the outcome for mother and child has been greatly enhanced. Likewise, GIFT and IVF programs have offered hope to those couples faced with infertility. For some, those medical advances are taken for granted, and their failure is greeted with anger and despair; while most couples are able to have 'normal' healthy children, not all are, and those faced with this are left to deal with grief, denial, anger, negotiation, depression and resolution (Kubler Ross). For couples where the woman has not become pregnant easily, or where she is pregnant in the setting of a previous miscarriage, stillbirth or adoption, the pregnancy becomes special.

For those with previous pregnancies, anxiety may be heightened about a repeated miscarriage, particularly at the same time into the pregnancy of the previous lost pregnancies, or about the infant's well-being. Where previous problems, such as cervical incompetence, can be treated, such treatment can bring some, but not necessarily total, relief. Where previous problems in the infant can be diagnosed (Down's syndrome, spina bifida), ultrasound and amniocentesis tests may be helpful but not necessarily totally curative. These women and their partners may or may not have adequately grieved over previous losses—a pregnancy now going to term can reawaken this grief. Feelings of anger and guilt can be directed at the infant, the self or the partner, with associated difficulties with bonding or with feelings of depression.

Those couples who conceive as a result of IVF/GIFT have often already endured years of feared infertility and invasive medical intervention. It would be understandable if these women were highly anxious, as Morse and Dennerstein (1985) found; other studies, however, have not found this association, and authors have commented on the reluctance of these women to admit to such anxiety (Haseltine et al 1985; Visser et al 1994). One woman said to me: 'I was a wreck, but I never let them [the medical profession] know ... I knew what they wanted to hear ... I wasn't about to put at risk something so important ...'. This anxiety was not relieved by the birth of a normal healthy child, but rather was intensified. A number of such women I have seen are overwhelmed—they have idealised infancy and motherhood and are prepared for the reality of neither.

With the increase in multiple pregnancies because of some medical procedures, this process is intensified—with increased guilt that they are not twice (or three) times as happy. For multiple pregnancies, where 1 (or more) infants is lost, the grief for this loss may be intense, even if the loss was at a very early gestation, and may affect the capacity to bond to the surviving infant(s). Such grief is often predominantly the domain of the woman; the fathers also grieve, but may be more pragmatic, and may often feel that they need to take on the role of supporter, putting aside their own grief. Perceived differing levels of grief, and the differing time taken to work through the process (usually faster in men) can put considerable strain on the marital relationship—added to the stress of parenthood where a child has survived, and little understood by well-meaning family and friends who are at a loss to understand the grief, when a healthy baby exists.

Special pregnancies—management issues

1. Ask whether conception occurred readily and, if not, if intervention was required. Assess the impact of this on the woman's and her partner's self-esteem. If the child is not the biological child of one or of either, this may have significant implications for the individual, for the couple, and for their reaction to and bonding with the child. Where psychiatric illness, particularly depression or anxiety, occurs in such a setting, these issues may need further discussion either with the individual or the couple. If these issues can be addressed prior to delivery (or conception), the path to parenthood may be a little smoother.
2. Ask about prior pregnancies: terminations, miscarriages, stillbirths or infants who died shortly after birth or who were adopted. Ask the couple how they dealt with this as individuals, and as a couple. Try to gauge at what stage the couple is in the grief process; each may be at different stages. Both are often aware of and frustrated by this; individual and/or couple counselling can be beneficial.
3. Counselling need not necessarily be intense or with a 'counsellor'. Allowing them to open up, and to have this grief acknowledged is, in itself, an important step towards resolution, and to minimising its effect on this and subsequent pregnancies.

Case example – 1
Nadia, 27, delivered a planned healthy son, David, after an uneventful pregnancy. She subsequently developed a postpartum psychosis, with suicidal depression requiring electroconvulsive therapy. While her

psychotic symptoms settled, a moderate level of depression persisted for many months, and was unresponsive to a variety of antidepressants in high doses. She appeared remote from, and almost fearful of, her child.

Nadia's husband, Graham, was supportive, and their prior relationship had been good. There was no previous or known family psychiatric history.

On one particular occasion, Nadia appeared to deteriorate dramatically, and her primary nurse noted that the admission of another woman to the ward had appeared to upset her. It transpired that it was not the woman who had upset her, but the woman's daughter, Amy.

Nadia spoke for the first time, to either staff or husband, of a previous pregnancy when she had been 16. The memory had been largely suppressed—but she recalled that she had given birth to a daughter, and had wanted to call the child Amy. Her parents, who had sent her to a convent for the pregnancy, had insisted that she have the child adopted. She had neither seen nor spoken to her daughter since.

The disclosure brought about initial deterioration—but gave meaning to her symptoms, and to the difficulties she had had with being David's mother. 'Amy' was in the way. Psychotherapy was able to help her gently disassemble the defences she had developed around the adoption, so that she could grieve, forgive herself and then tackle the task of again becoming a mother.

Case example – 2

Jean, 36, presented in pregnancy. She had been initially referred to a neurologist with a history of 'strange sensations' in her arms. No abnormality was found, and she was referred to a psychiatrist.

Jean had her first pregnancy at 17, as the result of a casual relationship. Although brought up in a Catholic family, she elected to have a termination, and felt she coped well with this. At 34, after having married Ted a year earlier, she had a boy with Down's syndrome who died from a congenital heart defect at 2 days. She reported that her first thought when told that he had Down's was 'God is punishing me'. She reported feeling very distressed, and that Ted was very supportive and stoic, but his being able to accept that it was 'God's will' that the child had died was irritating and abhorrent to her. Their relationship deteriorated, Jean saying that she felt unable to confide in Ted, and Ted reporting that he thought having another child would help.

Jean presented as anxious, but not depressed. She reported that when she was anxious, and apparently not with any particular precipitant, her hands would become 'cold and stiff'. The psychotherapist considered that this sounded like her memory of her dead child, but did not make the interpretation at this time.

Jean underwent several sessions of hypnotherapy. In one, she was asked to visualise the previous birth and subsequent events from the other side of a glass screen—as an onlooker. She was able to do so readily. At the next session, she presented agitated but elated. She related that while listening to a relaxation tape (part of her anxiety management strategy) she had a flashback to prior to the child's funeral, when her mother had insisted that she, Jean, view the body.

'I had seen Oliver alive and warm—I had wanted to remember him that way. But they showed me this shrivelled little *thing* . . . and made me touch it. I thought I would die . . . it was so cold and stiff.'

At this time the therapist made an interpretation of her symptoms, and Jean burst into tears; she allowed herself to release her anger and feel her pain. Subsequently there were no further 'strange sensations'. She was able to describe her feelings to her husband, and their relationship improved. She had a healthy girl, with no further psychiatric symptoms.

Denial of pregnancy

While uncommon, a number of cases where pregnancy has been denied, even right up to delivery, have been reported. This means of course that no antenatal care or preparation has occurred; there is also a suggestion that these babies are at a greater risk postpartum (Slayton & Soloft 1981; Mitchell & Davis 1984). Brezinka et al (1994) reviewed 27 such cases: 11 denied until delivery, 9 until 27–36 weeks and 7 until 21–26 weeks gestation. Infant outcomes were significantly poorer than would be expected in a 'normal' monitored pregnancy population, with 4 foetal deaths, 3 premature deliveries, an intra-uterine growth retardation and a concealed but discovered delivery. All the women had experienced significant stress (10 had separated from partners); just under half had a psychiatric diagnosis, including schizophrenia, major depression, personality disorder and mild mental retardation.

Denial of pregnancy seems to be a symptom of a heterogenous group of disorders and non-disorders. Consequentially, each case needs to be considered separately, with a full psychiatric assessment. Subsequent possible risk to the infant needs to be assessed in the setting of the diagnosis, current and on-going supports and the mother–infant relationship.

Case example

Lena, 15, was admitted for investigation of PV blood loss. In theatre, retained placental products were removed from her uterus. No history of pregnancy or of delivery had been given.

Lena was a plump, pleasant and somewhat shy girl, the middle of 3 children, all living at home with strict parents; the father was a minister of religion. It had been noticed that she had put on weight, but pregnancy had never been considered or suggested.

Lena herself claimed to be unaware of her pregnancy, describing intermittent bleeding and saying that her periods had always been irregular. She had had a sexual relationship occasionally with a boy in her class at school, of whom her parents mildly disapproved, largely because she was 'too young' to be seriously involved. Lena disliked school, and her intelligence was low average to borderline. There was no evidence of psychosis or depression.

The birth was described by Lena as being like 'gastro'; she had gone home early from school (her mother worked) and had laid down. When she thought that she was going to have an attack of diarrhoea, she went to the bathroom—and delivered. She related in a detached, matter-of-fact way that the baby was dead, so 'I cleaned up and buried it'. The corpse was found in the back garden. The autopsy report was not conclusive, and no charges were laid. Psychiatric follow-up was refused by Lena's father.

It was difficult to understand just what had happened in this case; Lena's low intelligence, her need for family approval and her strict upbringing are likely to have contributed to her denial of pregnancy— her subsequent detachment was of concern, and future pregnancies may well awaken the guilt and anger that she had been unable to face at the time.

Alcohol and drug abuse in pregnancy

The effect on the developing foetus of drugs, both prescribed and illicit, including alcohol and tobacco, has aroused increasing public and professional concern in recent times.

Nevertheless, a significant number of pregnant women use medication—in particular, non-narcotic analgesics and anti-emetics and also tobacco and alcohol (Rubin et al 1986). With the latter substances the incidence appears to be rising (Aftimos 1986; Litmen 1986).

Illicit drugs

It is estimated that 80–85% of narcotic and cocaine addicts are of child-bearing age. Although the incidence of narcotic use in pregnancy in Australia between 1978–82 was thought to be as low as 0.06% (Oats et al 1984), which is less than the 3–5% American estimates, an increase had occurred in the number of pregnant addicts during the 1980s. Well recognised foetal complications include intra-uterine death, infection in up to 60%, prematurity in 14–27%, and growth retardation with a poorer prognosis than babies of non-addicts (Zelson et al 1971; Stern 1985; Klenka 1986; Tylden et al 1986; Alroomi et al 1988; Verloove-Vanhack et al 1988; Wilson et al 1979).

Cocaine increases the likelihood of spontaneous abortion with placental abruption (MacGregor et al 1987; Critchley et al 1988).

In neonates the neonatal abstinence syndrome occurs in 7% (Klenka 1986; Tylden et al 1986), and performance is thought to be decreased on perceptual tests (Stern 1985; Tylden et al 1986). There is an increased mortality also (Klenka 1986). In older children, performance on cognition and perception is considerably lower, with behavioural disturbances and neuromotor abnormalities (Wilson et al 1979).

Maternal complications are also common: 40–50% of these women develop anaemia or a variety of infections, and up to 75% report depression. Poor nutrition, less antenatal care and inadequate sleep are also common (Stern 1985).

Use of marijuana in pregnancy is often associated with an intake of tobacco and alcohol and the specific effects of each are difficult to delineate. Neonatal effects are dose dependent, and an increase in prematurity and growth retardation is reported. Neurological and morphological abnormalities are controversial (Aftimos 1986).

Alcohol

A much higher incidence of alcohol use in pregnancy compared to illicit drugs is noted (Sokol 1981; Rosett & Weiner 1981; Stern 1984). Since 1968 the gender ratio for alcohol intake of those less than 40 years of age has altered from a ratio of 3 males:1 female to 2:1 in 1982 (Aftimos 1986; Beary & Merry 1986).

The foetal effects of alcohol have been documented since Greek and Roman mythology (Warner & Rossett 1975) and have received a higher profile since the foetal alcohol syndrome was described by Jones and Smith in 1973. Prenatal and postnatal growth retardation, cranio-facial abnormalities and CNS dysfunction are features of this syndrome. In the neonate a disturbed sleeping pattern is noted (Rosett & Weiner 1981; Weiner et al 1983). The amount of alcohol intake required to cause this syndrome is uncertain. There are disparities in the definition of 'light', 'moderate' and 'heavy' drinking. Questionnaires have low return rates and are often retrospective, and thus forgetfulness and denial play a part (Weiner et al 1983; Barrison et al 1985). Averages are not useful as in some instances alcohol may act as an acute fetotoxin (Kline et al 1980) and as few as two drinks a week are associated with an increased incidence of spontaneous abortion (Kline et al 1980). One study suggests that heavy drinking prior to conception may be deleterious even if abstinence is observed throughout pregnancy (Barrison et al 1985).

Unlike smokers, nearly all women who drink reduce their alcohol intake in pregnancy. Condon and Hilton (1988) reported that 100% of women in their study reduced their alcohol intake, and noted the decrease to be directly related to strong antenatal attachment. The ambivalent mother was more likely to continue drinking. Kwok et al (1983) also report a more significant reduction in alcohol than nicotine, with 99% of those who consumed alcohol in pregnancy doing so only occasionally, whereas the smokers continued to smoke throughout.

Prescribed drugs

The effect of psychotropic drugs in pregnancy is reviewed in Chapter 8.

Alcohol and drug abuse in pregnancy—management issues

Management of women who abuse alcohol and/or drugs in pregnancy needs to be considered from the point of view of:

1. current physical health;
2. current emotional health;
3. on-going risks to self;
4. current foetal state;
5. on-going risk to foetus.

Women who attend obstetric care may not be prepared to seek help for their dependency. Denial, fear, guilt and the possibility of stigma contribute to this. Management of these women to date has been stigmatised and overmedicalised. Emphasis has traditionally been given to the woman as a nurturer and mother. This approach fails to view the woman as an individual in her own right, and does not take into account the aetiology and consequences of drug use. Illicit-drug users are more likely to have a disturbed family background, with features such as: no suitable parental model, incest, rape and family violence. Self-esteem is likely to be compromised by prostitution, guilt regarding the drug abuse, lack of a partner, or a non-supportive partner and inadequate social supports. In this setting, pregnancy will be an added stress. Helping the woman gain understanding of her past, and establish ways of being in control of her present and future, will enhance self-esteem and replace the need for drugs.

Trust may not be readily given to medical staff for fear of exposure. High anxiety is likely to lead to increased drug intake, leading to financial pressures and further guilt feelings towards the unborn child (Stern 1985; Tylden et al 1986). The arrival of a child who is ill will enhance the guilt. Guilt and depression as well as physical illness in mother and child will impair bonding and the capacity for the woman to mother. A cycle of failure and further lowering of self-esteem is likely to perpetuate drug use rather than enhance motherhood. Intervention through pregnancy and following delivery may need to be intensive—and long-term. It may also not be accepted, even when offered.

Case example

Irene, 32, and her 4-day-old son, Liam, were transferred to a mother-baby unit from an antenatal ward, where concern had been raised about her level of anxiety. Irene denied any problems, but was observed to be tremulous, worsening when she was required to handle the child. Liam was thought to be 'jittery' and 'look odd'; the paediatricians were noncommittal at this time.

Irene became increasingly agitated, claiming that it was being in hospital that was causing her problem. She discharged herself against medical advice. Two days later she was admitted to an orthopaedic ward of a general hospital, having fractured her pelvis in a fall. Her blood-alcohol reading at the time was 0.25.

Irene and her husband, also a heavy drinker, refused to accept that her drinking was a problem. Irene became angry and defensive at suggestions that her child might have foetal alcohol syndrome. Protective services were involved at this stage in view of the possible risk to Liam; their involvement forced her (although reluctantly) to attend a rehabilitation centre; the long-term success remains to be evaluated.

The birth

Through the latter part of pregnancy, the woman becomes more focused on the birth. Current trends have directed the focus towards demedicalising birth, emphasising the naturalness of both birth and pregnancy, and the importance of physical and psychological well-being in making birth less of a medical procedure. While this allows the woman a sense of control, it does not prepare her for the reality; birth is for most extremely painful, and current Australian medical practice involves a (relatively) high level of intervention. As a result, for some women the experience is unexpectedly traumatic. Not only must they deal with the physical stresses and changes of the postpartum and the overwhelming realisation of the dependency and responsibility of this new child but, as well, there may be a sense of failure.

The process of birth, for some women, becomes idealised. Self-esteem may be tied closely to the idea of the pregnancy and birth being normal, the normality reinforcing a sense of achievement and status as a woman. Medical intervention may be regarded as her own failure, both physically and psychologically; there may be anger at herself, and also at the treating clinicians. Inadequate discussion and explanation and the expectation of passive acquiescence by many medical professionals only heightens this process—separating further the reality from the ideal, and emphasising the powerlessness of the woman.

Some studies (Dennerstein et al 1989) have found stress related to the delivery process to be associated with postpartum depression. In a literature review Fisher et al (1990) concluded that Caesarean section was associated with an increased psychological morbidity, but not with an increase in depression. The issue of needing to be in control was particularly highlighted.

Birth may present a special problem for women with schizophrenia. If they are psychotic, they may be unaware of the symptoms of labour, and are more likely to be unco-operative with labour staff—who usually have little psychiatric experience (Spielvogel & Wile 1986). Pregnant women with schizophrenia need close monitoring, particularly at term; if they are psychotic it is preferable that they are admitted, unless living with supportive families.

The birth—management issues

1. Throughout pregnancy encourage a focus on the outcome rather than the process of birth, that is, a healthy infant and mother, and on planning for dealing with the reality of caring for a young infant.

2. During the birth process, keep the woman and her partner fully informed of progress (or the lack of), and wherever possible give clear explanations for any needed interventions, allowing input and questions. These explanations may need to be repeated and reworded; the couple is generally not medically trained and in a crisis, anxiety may interfere with comprehension. The fear of the unknown and the loss of power are crucial issues throughout birth, and can be minimised in most situations by emphatic listening and patient explanations. Many complaints (including litigious ones) associated with childbirth are related to this, rather than to the intervention or outcome itself.

3. All women and their partners should be given the opportunity to 'debrief'—to talk about their experiences and ask questions. Some, who have not dealt with these issues, may request to do so later. Spending time going through the notes and explaining procedures can be beneficial even weeks or months later. Issues pertaining to previous births may arise in subsequent pregnancies; dealing with this early may prevent later anxiety.

Case example

Corinne, 29, had had 3 children, each delivered by Caesarean section due to cephalopelvic disproportion. The initial Caesarean had occurred

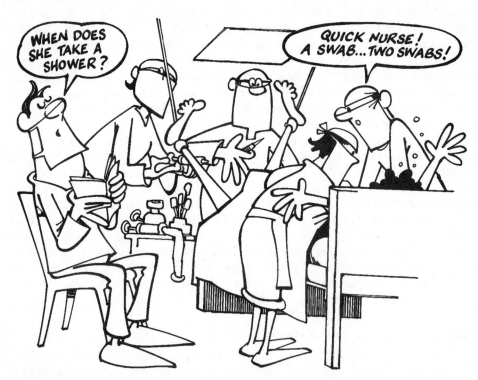

The woman ... and her partner ... become more focused on the 'demedicalised' birth

after a trial of labour with failure to progress and foetal distress. The subsequent Caesareans had been elective.

Corinne described wanting children since her early teenage years. Although she had been a successful nurse, and knew more about the birth process than most women, she had felt that childbirth (rather than rearing) was the most important experience a woman could have. It was the one thing she could do that her brothers could not; throughout her childhood she felt that she had battled (and lost) against them for her father's attention.

After the first birth, Corinne described being in a state of shock. She felt she had 'failed'; after many months and discussions with several obstetricians she accepted that she would never be able to give birth vaginally. She subsequently resolved to have the 'perfect Caesarean'.

After both subsequent births, Corinne was disappointed with the experience and became significantly depressed. Neither experience had met with her expectations; her expectations of immediate attachment and powerful emotion were unrealistic, and did not take account of the effects of pain and analgesics—and of the emotional and physical demands of a young infant. Brief psychotherapy focused on issues of self-esteem, refocusing her on her role of mothering, at which she was very competent. The depression resolved slowly, without medication.

CHAPTER 4

Childhood reflections

New parents do not begin their new role with a clean slate. As Fraiberg et al (1980) have put it so well—in every nursery, there are ghosts. While for some parents these ghosts may rarely be intrusive, for others the arrival of an infant arouses issues from childhood. An infant is a constant reminder of having been a child, and of the parenting experienced then. In negotiating the transition to parenthood, experiences from childhood, and the relationship particularly with parents, will affect the quality, attitudes and consistency achieved. Combined with genetic influences, childhood experiences will have shaped the personality, and may also have contributed to the emergence of psychiatric illness prior to having had a child. For some women, having a child of their own will be a stressful and traumatic reminder of the past, and will highlight personal difficulties.

Relationship to parents

For some women, the arrival of a child brings them closer to their own parents, and enables them to be more understanding of the difficulties their parents had faced. This process requires a maturity in the negotiations of the role changes, and presumes minimal emotional scarring from the childhood relationship. This is not always the case and such scarring predisposes to psychiatric illness.

A number of researchers have documented links between the relationship to parents in childhood and the later development of psychiatric illness. Family pathology in the past had been considered aetiological in schizophrenia (Lidz 1958) but is now viewed more as a potential stress and trigger of episodes.

Rogosch et al (1992), looking at parenting attitudes in women with schizophrenia and major mood disorders, found negative attitudes associated with the recollection of lack of maternal involvement, and that this was also linked with current emotional support and self-esteem.

Studies on families with a member with anorexia nervosa have identified increased psychopathology in the parents, in particular pathological attitudes and behaviour related to weight, that appear to transmit themselves from generation to generation and that are not apparently genetic (Kalucy et al 1977).

Brown and Harris (1978) in the Camberwell study found a link between the loss of the mother before the age of 11 and later depression; Parker (1979) found, in a predominantly female sample, that those with neurotic depression were more likely to report maternal over-protective and less parental care. A bipolar sample, however, did not differ from controls.

Researchers looking specifically at postpartum depression have also looked at establishing a link with parental relationship.

The importance of these developmental relationships remains unclear. Dennerstein et al (1989) found that an unhappy childhood, the level of assistance of the woman's father postpartum and the woman's mother's reaction to the birth to be important. Kumar and Robson (1984) found early separation from the father (not the mother) and current difficulties in the relationship with the mother were associated.

In the clinical in-patient and out-patient population I see, issues with parents from the past frequently re-emerge postpartum. For some, this may be related to a history of abuse, but for others it is perhaps a more subtle, but nevertheless longstanding and destructive relationship that may well have begun from infancy, and be related to the new mother's own mother's background, genetics, personality and/or illness. Rohner and Rohner (1980) described how rejection as a child affected the woman's development, and then predisposed her to rejection of her own child—a potentially spiralling negative cycle. Violence in families may also be inter-generational (Carroll 1977).

Beside dealing with the past, the new parents must adjust to being simultaneously children and parents, and the grandparents must renegotiate their relationship to their child, their child's spouse and their child's child. Where roles have been unclear, boundaries blurred and self-worth uncertain, such negotiations are hazardous.

The arrival of a child may in some cases re-involve parents who had been largely excluded from the couple's life. The re-involvement may be due to social and cultural pressures on either the new parents or the grandparents. Attitudes to the child may differ significantly, and may be the source of on-going friction where the grandparents are unable to accept the limitations of their role or the new parents to assert theirs.

The most frequent problem seen is the relationship between the new mother and her own mother. Some women idealise the role of motherhood, and are disappointed when their mother fails to live up to this, and add this to their own expectations of themselves to do better for this child than was done for them.

Mothers are often criticised for inadequate care and protection (particularly where women have a history of childhood sexual abuse) and for being unable to form a close relationship with their daughters. Some daughters experience these same difficulties with their own daughters. They feel unable to ask their own mothers for help or advice and, if they do, fear ridicule and the perpetuation of a power struggle where they still continue to feel the child in the relationship. Such confrontations are often avoided, but where grandparents are relied on for child care—for financial reasons or because of a greater fear of strangers caring for the child—this may not be possible.

Issues between the new mother and her in-laws, or between the father and his own parents or in-laws may also exist. Issues of non-acceptance that pre-date the birth of the child can improve—but for a new parent lacking in self-esteem, already feeling a failure, the situation may actually worsen, or be perceived to do so.

Relationship to parents—management issues

1. Women with postpartum psychiatric disorders require family and social support; they not only have an infant for whom to care, but also an illness with which to deal. Care for the infant is not readily available out of hours and families, where available, are heavily relied upon. Before suggesting that a parent or in-law be involved, or if they are already involved, assess how comfortable the woman and her partner are with this arrangement. In a crisis it may be essential but, longer term, it may create as many problems as it helps.

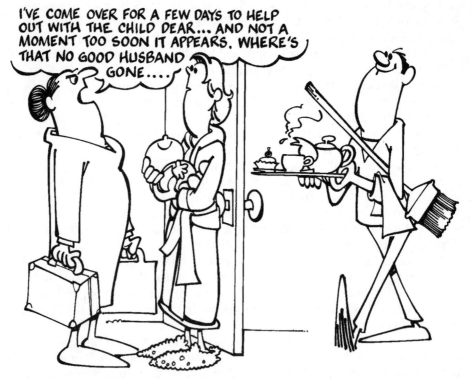

Before suggesting a parent or in-law be involved, assess how comfortable the woman and her partner are with this arrangement

2. Remember to ask the woman about her relationship with her parents, and in particular how she feels this has shaped her own attitudes to parenting. Are her expectations of herself in relation to her own mother reasonable? If she is motivated not to behave as her own parent did, she may require strategies to help herself. Under stress, it is often instinctive to resort to tactics used by the role model (usually her own parent). I saw one woman, who was physically abused as a child, resolve never to smack her child; yet, when he cried constantly for several hours, she hit a 4-week-old infant on several occasions. Such 'failures' can be a shock (and in this case dangerous) and can add to the guilt and lowered self-esteem. It can also be used as a turning point in understanding and accepting one's parent's limitations.

3. For some parents, individual work over some time is needed to help them work through their past relationship with their parents, to enable them to deal with their partners in the present, and for them to come to terms with their own strengths and weaknesses as a parent. In some cases, the clinician seeing the grandparent may be important; be careful not to negotiate this until the woman is well enough to deal with issues arising from such an interview. Family relationships and secrets can be very powerful; where there is the suggestion of a very disturbed family, the involvement of an experienced therapist is recommended.

Case example – 1

Bernice, 25, had had a very close, confiding relationship with her mother, Angela, who had died after a prolonged illness 8 years earlier. Bernice had been engaged at the time, and had married her husband, Steve, a year later. After the birth of her first child (a girl) when she was 20, she developed a panic disorder. She had been reluctant to take medication, but finally agreed, and her symptoms settled. At age 23, she had another child, a boy, with no recurrence, although she described herself as being generally anxious. After the birth of another girl a year later, her symptoms re-emerged, with increased severity, to the extent that she became agoraphobic. She rarely left the house, being able to do so only after medication or alcohol, neither of which she liked, as she associated both with her mother's illness (Angela had had liver disease, but this was hepatic and not alcohol-related).

Although Bernice's symptoms improved on tricyclic antidepressants, they did not resolve. It became apparent that periodic episodes of deterioration were closely related to marital conflict. Her husband was not agreeable to counselling, and Bernice did not tell him that she was continuing to see a psychiatrist.

While many issues arose in individual counselling, the most pertinent related to Bernice's attitude to her mother, and how this affected her attitude to Steve. Bernice experienced great anger—and guilt—regarding her mother. Angela had been ill and largely bed-ridden since Bernice was 8 years old. Bernice, as the only daughter, had had to assume responsibility for the care of her mother as well as for the house and looking after her 3 brothers and father. Prior to her mother's death, her father had separated from Angela, and Bernice and Steve had had to move in with her. Bernice had felt torn between caring for Angela, and wanting to be young and enjoying her relationship with Steve and planning their wedding. Angela's death meant that the latter was postponed, and was consequently a sombre affair. By dying, Angela also 'missed out' on grandchildren, and was unavailable to Bernice for advice and support.

As a result, Bernice had very powerful emotions of anger that horrified her and which she was unable to face. That anger which did surface was largely directed at Steve, for preventing her from adequately caring for, or even saving, her mother. The panic symptoms seemed to represent the panic she felt when faced with the guilt that threatened to overwhelm her.

Behavioural therapy, with flooding techniques—forcing her to sit through an increasing hierarchy of anxiety-provoking situations—helped her panic symptoms, but she then became depressed. It was while she was depressed that she was able to look at her relationship with her mother—and then at that with her daughters to whom she had had difficulties being close.

Case example – 2

Marion, 35, was admitted with her 2-month-old daughter. She was no longer able to cope at home, where she feared she might harm her 3-year-old son. She described him as having regressed since his sister's birth, throwing tantrums, defecating on the floor and bed-wetting.

In hospital, Marion was irritable, reluctant to care for her child, demanding, and critical of staff. Her husband, Tom, was quietly despairing and passive. He described a previously good relationship that had deteriorated since their son's birth, and had worsened further in the previous month.

Marion had no past or family psychiatric history, but described an unhappy childhood where, whatever she did, it was never good enough for her parents. She saw her mother as dominating and opinionated; there had been minimal contact for a number of years. Marion considered Tom's mother also critical and unhelpful, and resented the time that Tom spent with her (usually once a week on the way home from work).

Through couple and individual work, it became evident that Marion was angry at her mother's failure to care for and love her as a child, and that she was recreating the pattern with her own children. She had an idealised picture of what a mother/grandparent should be, and Tom's mother could never hope to live up to this. Therapy helped her initially evaluate her expectations, and then look to herself and her marital relationship for satisfaction, rather than blaming others and not taking responsibility for herself.

Personality

While geneticists argue that most, if not all, of one's personality is predetermined by biology, there is evidence that childhood events, particularly major childhood trauma, can have a significant effect on the development of the personality (Wheeler & Walton 1987).

Certain personality styles may render a woman more prone to a depressive illness, and may also be affected by the illness. People presenting with depression can appear dependent and inadequate, or other previously present traits may be markedly accentuated. These characteristics may no longer create a problem when the illness has been resolved.

There is evidence, however, that certain premorbid personality features are associated with an increased risk of depression. These include dependency, obsessionality, neuroticism and high interpersonal sensitivity. Boyce et al (1991) found the latter 2 characteristics to be a risk factor for the onset and recurrence of postpartum depression, whether or not there was a past history of depression. Other researchers have found an association between postpartum depression and neuroticism (Pitt 1968; Meares et al 1976; Watson et al 1984); Kumar and Robson (1984) found an association only with antenatal depression. These women frequently have a history of high anxiety and difficulties coping with stress; the baby may represent a constant and excessive stress.

Obsessional women may also become depressed (Klein & Depue 1985), particularly in the first few months, when routines may vary and when a mother is required to be flexible. Much anxiety can be experienced by these women. Previous rules and patterns, and preconceived ideas about motherhood are challenged; for some, this can lead to decompensation and depression.

Women with antisocial or borderline personality traits may experience a number of difficulties providing a consistent and supportive environment for their children. Many borderline patients have significant issues from childhood, such as abuse and deprivation, with which to deal. Alcohol and substance abuse will have effects on them, on their ability to form a relationship with the child, and on their capacity to safely care for their child. Where there is no supportive partner or family, protective/welfare services are likely to become involved.

Personality—management issues

1. When assessing the role of personality, it is essential to consider the lifelong pattern of behaviour, and not just that in relation to the illness; depressed or psychotic women may present quite differently to their normal selves. For women who have had a chronic, perhaps untreated,

illness after the birth of an older child, it may be difficult for the woman or her partner to recall the premorbid personality. In women conceiving at a very young age, this also presents a special difficulty.

2. Whether 'genetic' or not, particular features of the personality may need to be addressed to help the women resolve the acute symptoms; obsessional women who feel out of control can benefit from behavioural therapy and rational emotive techniques. Simple things, such as priority lists and emphasising the positives of doing one or more tasks, rather than the failure of not completing them all, can assist day-to-day life. Alcohol and substance abuse need to be treated as problems in their own right, addressing issues of safety. Like most depressed people, women with high neuroticism and interpersonal sensitivity lack self-esteem; individual and group work can address this. Skills such as learning to be assertive may also be of benefit.

3. People with personality disorders can be difficult to deal with. If, as the clinician, you experience anger and frustration towards a patient, it is important to try and understand why—what is it that this patient is doing to elicit this response? Patients who are demanding and unappreciative and who fail to respond to therapy are frequently disliked; but what is it that they are feeling, and how much of this is their 'fault'? Women with postpartum psychiatric disorders, who have had a deprived back-ground, may be acting out their own childhood, with you as their parent; they may expect to be rejected, because they feel unlovable. As the clinician, it is important to try to be consistent and caring, but with firm boundaries.

Case example – 1

Hilary, 38, an English school teacher, had been married for 2 years and had come to Australia with her husband when she was in the early stages of pregnancy. Since arriving, she had been irritable, anxious and fought frequently with her husband, James. After the birth of their son, Callum, she became increasingly depressed, and her anger turned on the infant whom she claimed she had never wanted, and whom she held responsible for all her problems: 'If not for him I could return home [to England]'.

Hilary was admitted because she no longer wished to care for Callum, and James had become increasingly concerned about it. Throughout the admission she cared for Callum reluctantly, and was taciturn and sullen. Staff were unable to form a relationship with her, and experienced anger at her rejection of Callum, a delightful, happy baby.

Initially as an in-patient, and then as an out-patient, Hilary had trials on a number of antidepressants with no improvement. James filed for divorce—and for custody. The psychiatric report at the time indicated Hilary had antisocial personality traits and this contributed to James attaining custody.

Two years after Callum's birth, on a new antidepressant, Hilary made a full recovery. There was not—and never had been—a history of antisocial personality; the anger and instability were part of her depressive illness. The interpretation of antisocial behaviour was related to the inability to obtain a history from anyone other than her husband, and to the frustration and anger experienced by staff. Hilary didn't regain custody of Callum.

Case example – 2

Nina, 27, had a history of rigid obsessionality and high levels of anxiety. Her house was ordered and clean, and her life run to routine.

She had an ambivalent relationship with her mother, whom she saw frequently, but who made her increasingly agitated, 'because I can see I'm just like her ... and I don't want to be'.

Nina's pregnancy was planned; her first disappointment and feelings of failure related to her requiring a Caesarean due to failure to progress. She then experienced considerable difficulty breastfeeding: her anxiety prevented her letting down the milk, and her tension communicated to her infant who appeared reluctant to attach; she perceived this as rejection.

In the first months postpartum, Nina's anxiety escalated. She became increasingly disorganised and despaired of this, frantically doing housework at odd hours of the night in an attempt to keep her world in control.

Therapy initially required medication, to control her depressive symptoms, and time. Time and anxiety management techniques, combined with parent education and work on her expectations, helped her daily management. By 6 months postpartum her infant had settled into a routine, and she declined any offer of further individual therapy.

Childhood sexual abuse (CSA)

A significantly higher proportion of abused than non-abused women suffer psychiatric disorder. Mullen and colleagues (1988) estimated that 20% of women who had been sexually abused as children had a psychiatric illness, compared with 6.3% of the non-abused female population having a depressive illness in the 3-year study period. A study of female psychiatric in-patients and out-patients has found over 60% have a history of abuse (Bryer et al 1987; Surrey et al 1990). In comparison to general practice patients, psychiatric patients reported rates 2 or 3 times greater than the general practice patients (Palmer et al 1993).

The nature of the link is uncertain. CSA is often associated with physical abuse, emotional abuse, neglect and other signs of a dysfunctional, chaotic household. It has been suggested that these factors may be as important as the nature of the CSA in determining later adult psychopathology (Beitchman et al 1992; Mullen et al 1993). Such psychopathology includes depression (Beitchman et al 1992; Bifulco et al 1991), eating disorders (Mullen et al 1993), substance abuse, personality disorders and disturbances (Beitchman et al 1992; Tong et al 1978) and sexual dysfunction (Hyde 1984). Difficulties in relationships and in parenting have been reported and are common in clinical practice, although little relevant research appears to have been published with respect to this, or to psychiatric disorders developing postpartum (Cole et al 1992).

As with many other psychiatric disorders, CSA appears to be a risk factor for postpartum psychiatric disorder (Buist & Barnett, in press). This is not difficult to understand. The arrival of a child presents the woman with an infant as vulnerable and as needy as she herself may feel.

A history of CSA is associated with low self-esteem—thrown into a new role, this can be worsened.

Women affected by CSA are more likely to have negative views of their mothers and fathers and have difficulty in relationships with men; they are thus less likely to have supportive families and marital relationships. The delivery itself may be perceived as a physical assault (often involving a male obstetrician) and procedures such as forceps can induce flashbacks. The sex of the child may be an issue—a male seen as a future perpetrator, a girl as someone in need of protection that the mother may be uncertain she can provide.

In Waldby's study (1984), 80% of women felt their relationship to their own children had been affected by CSA, describing over-protection, emotional and disciplinary problems and postpartum depression. Researchers looking at parenting issues have found women with a history of CSA to be less confident and to feel out of control as parents (Cole et al 1992), to have a tendency to rely on children as supports (Burkett 1991) and to promote (excessive) autonomy to the extent of parent–child role reversal (Cole & Woolger 1989; Burkett 1991). The observation of the permeability of inter-generational boundaries raises particular concerns given the increased incidence of inter-generational incest in these families.

In the in-patient unit at the Mercy Hospital, more than half the women admitted have a history of CSA; this is a little less than some studies (Bryer et al 1987; Surrey et al 1990) but it must be remembered that some survivors choose not to have children. These admissions tend to be longer and more staff-intensive than those of women without a history of CSA. Many of these women have not previously disclosed their abuse and have had no, or minimal, counselling. The birth of their child brings memories of the past to the surface; issues involving their parents, their partners and their infants are mixed together in women who are often in many ways still negotiating adolescence or earlier life stages. These issues are not easily dealt with: these women can be difficult, angry, demanding, labile or suicidal. They are extremely distressed and needy, and often have little to give to an infant. Some of the work can begin postpartum, but it often needs to continue for months or years subsequently.

Childhood sexual abuse—management issues

1. A history of sexual abuse in women with psychiatric illness is common; the treating health professional needs to ask if the woman has experienced CSA. This is best done when some rapport has been developed, perhaps on the second or third interview. It may need to be asked again, later in treatment, if symptoms, behaviours or 'throw away lines' alert the therapist to the possibility. Ask, do not suggest, and ask only if you are able to deal with an affirmative answer. This means acknowledging what is being said, acknowledging the pain and in no way trivialising the issue or blaming the woman.

2. An affirmative answer does not necessarily mean that the woman needs to, or wishes to, deal with the issues of abuse. It may not be relevant or appropriate, or the woman may not be ready.

3. The offer of help to deal with the issues of abuse in therapy is important, but the acute symptoms need to have settled, and where possible the health professional should be able to offer long-term follow-up. Where this is not possible, such as in an in-patient setting, this should be made clear from the start, and termination of treatment of the woman should be approached gradually, while handing over to the out-patient therapist.

4. This woman may need long-term supports and intervention; so may her partner, and her child.

Case example – 1

Ellen, 29, was transferred to a mother-baby unit from an obstetric hospital where she had delivered her first child 4 days prior. During labour she had become excessively distressed and had required sedation. In the days after delivery her moods swung violently, and she appeared disorientated and confused at times. On the day prior to transfer she had found herself (in pyjamas) in a shopping centre some distance from the hospital, with no memory of how she had got there. A general medical work-up was negative.

Ellen was living in a de facto relationship, and had worked in a variety of jobs. She had seen a counsellor briefly following a termination of pregnancy at 16, and a marriage guidance counsellor prior to her first marriage break-up, in her early 20s. Her father had a history of heavy alcohol use and her mother was a heavy user of minor tranquillisers. Ellen said that she was 'close' to them both, although her childhood had been 'pretty unhappy'.

Ellen appeared significantly depressed. She was reluctant to remain in hospital but was terrified of leaving, although she was unable to say why. At times her mood became slightly elevated, particularly when her parents visited, and she was noted to be disinhibited and inappropriate at these times, as well as in her interactions with male staff.

Two weeks after admission, Ellen broke down one evening, screaming and saying that she wanted to kill herself. She subsequently disclosed, for the first time, memories of CSA which had first been brought to her consciousness by feeling powerless in stirrups and being confronted by an obstetrician with forceps. Her history of CSA, involving her father, uncle and her two brothers, had begun at 6, continued until she was 12, and had involved horrific abuse, including violence and sadism.

Ellen deteriorated and required a prolonged hospitalisation. The flooding memories terrified her, making her feel vile, worthless and suicidal. She was unable to assume any care of her child for some weeks. She was, however, able to establish a supportive trusting relationship with her therapist, and it was from this that she gained strength and was able, finally and gradually, to return home. The risk of suicide and acting-out remained prominent; the long- and short-term risks to the child were significant.

Case example – 2

Brenda, 35, presented with depression after the birth of her second child, a girl. Her son was aged 4, and she felt that she had coped well after his birth. She now described herself as feeling overwhelmed. Her husband, a labourer, although practically supportive, was not attuned to psychological needs and appeared to have little understanding of his articulate and highly intelligent wife.

Brenda's depression worsened, despite high doses of anti-depressants, to the extent that she feared she would harm her child. She was admitted to a mother-baby unit, where she was noted to be a very caring and protective mother, who would not allow anyone else to assume care of her infant. At times she appeared frightened by the responsibility, and requested a nurse to sit with her.

Brenda's parents had separated when she was 10. Her father, a pharmacist, lived interstate, and she rarely saw her mother. She was reluctant to discuss them. She had had a number of brief liaisons; her marriage was her only long-term relationship. She had seen a psychologist intermittently over a number of years but was unable to say why, apart from a comment that 'the counsellor said I must have been abused'. When asked whether she had been, she was evasive.

On a weekend leave, when her husband had 'forcibly persuaded' her to have sexual intercourse, she returned to the unit in the middle of the night, tearful and distressed. Over the course of some weeks, she disclosed extensive sadomasochistic abuse by a circle of her father's friends. During this time of disclosure she was suicidal, and unable to care for her infant. She refused to disclose this to her husband for fear that he would reject her. She was, however, highly intelligent and highly motivated; she responded dramatically to Eye Movement Desensitisation and Reprocessing (EMDR) and, although counselling continued after discharge, her mood lifted without antidepressants and her relationship with her daughter, although over-protective, was warm and appropriate.

These cases are typical of the women admitted who have a history of CSA. A number of factors alert to the possibility of CSA (although they are in no way, in themselves, conclusive):

- a history of unstable relationships;
- a history of job instability;
- a suggestion of unfulfilled potential;
- alcohol and drug use in the family;
- dissociative states;
- disinhibited, flirtatious behaviour, more suggestive of inappropriate boundaries, not associated with mania.

The longer stay, and the period of deterioration with inability to care for the child, are also very typical. Management is intensive and time-consuming; but if interventions at this time can in any way improve the outlook for the mother and her relationship to her infant, and thus the infant's well-being, it is time well spent.

CHAPTER 5

Partners becoming parents

Transition to parenthood

Like other life stages, the transition to parenthood is one which can be difficult. Although pregnancy helps to prepare the future parents over a number of months, the arrival of the infant brings a sudden change in lifestyle and roles. In most cases, the changes occur simultaneously to *two* people, not just one. The arrival may have quite different effects on different individuals within a couple, and reactions and adaptation may occur at different rates. The parents may have already—although not necessarily fully or successfully—negotiated the changes required to adapt to being a couple. Now they face changes in this relationship and the forming of new ones. These will be most marked with the first child, but each family addition brings about further changes.

Throughout pregnancy, the woman tends to become introspective. Although her partner can feel the foetus move also, it is she who is primarily aware of it. This frequently continues into the postpartum months; one woman described it as if she had 'fallen out of love with my husband, and in love with my baby'. The baby demands a lot of physical attention and time—the time that the woman previously had for herself, and for her relationship with her partner. She may be tired, irritable, resentful and feel that she achieves less than previously. Poor preparation for, and understanding of, these potential experiences can lead to anger and frustration, often taken out on the partner.

The partner, on the other hand, may be dealing with his own issues of accepting and dealing with the responsibility of being the sole (even if temporary) breadwinner. Many couples are moving house, or have perhaps moved, or renovated with the impending need for increased space; this often creates extra financial stress for the male partner, and extra responsibility for the woman.

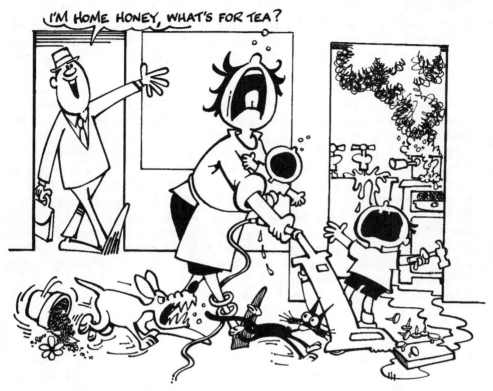

Like other life stages, the transition to parenthood can be difficult

The partner may feel excluded, rejected and unloved; the infant in the first few months gives little in the interaction and, if breastfed, the role of the father is minimised. In addition, sexual frequency and satisfaction is frequently diminished. Fischman et al's survey (1986) of postpartum couples revealed that sexual frequency had decreased in 84% of couples at 4 months and 60% of couples at 12 months after the birth. Women reported that physical discomfort, their dissatisfaction with their body shape, and fatigue contributed to this. Breastfeeding, and its necessarily lowered oestrogen and progesterone levels, also contribute to significantly decreased libido (Alder & Bancroft 1988).

Psychiatric morbidity in the father

Paternal psychiatric illness can be considered in a number of ways:
1. the man has a history of psychiatric illness prior to the birth of the child; and/or
2. the man develops a psychiatric illness associated with the birth of his child; and/or
3. the man develops a psychiatric illness associated with his wife's postpartum psychiatric illness.

Past history

If the father has a clear psychiatric history his illness needs to be treated, as appropriate. The stress of a child may, for fathers as well as for mothers, precipitate relapse. Ideally, all fathers should be included with their partners in discussions of expectations of parenthood and in ways of minimising stress. This is particularly so where fathers have a history of psychiatric disorder. For the woman, her husband's illness will be an added stress with which she has to deal, and may diminish his capacity to support her and be available for child care.

Where both partners have a history of psychiatric disorder, the issues of the couple's capacity to care for the child may need to be assessed and addressed. Up to 80% of spouses of people with schizophrenia have a psychiatric disorder (Fowler & Tsuang 1975; Alanen & Kinnunen 1975; Parnas 1988). The stability of the disorder in both parents needs to be monitored, and a clear safety net for the child established. Late pregnancy and the early postpartum period is an especially critical time. Where both parents have a significant, chronic illness, the long-term care of the child needs to be considered. This care may include:

- regular monitoring of parental medication;
- regular home visits;
- child care;
- home supports;
- protective services.

For parents in whom the illness is chronic, these supports may need to be longstanding.

Case example

Stefan, 50, had a long history of schizophrenia with multiple brief admissions in a number of different capital cities. He had extensive paranoid delusions that had settled but did not fully resolve on medication; he was, however, noncompliant with medication. Twenty years earlier, during an admission, he had met Barbara, 5 years his junior, and had married her shortly after. She had been diagnosed as having an anxiety disorder and had had no further admissions or follow-up until aged 45. At this time, school authorities alerted protective services about their 12-year-old child, leading to the involvement of the local GP and subsequent certification of both parents. Barbara at this time was diagnosed as having schizophrenia. This was later amended to 'folie à deux', a psychotic disorder occurring only under the influence of her husband. The child was grossly regressed, being illiterate and incontinent; it appears that her mother had managed to evade professional involvement for 12 years by changing schools and keeping the child at home. Barbara herself had not left the house in 5 years. Stefan, in this time, had had 2 brief admissions; at no time had his capacity to parent been considered.

With histories such as these, the welfare of the child *must* be considered paramount. Protective services should have been involved early in the postnatal period. An assessment of parenting ability should certainly be done in the hospital at the time of birth. Admission to a mother-baby hospital or unit may be required for more extensive evaluation. Follow-up, where there are any concerns, needs to be vigilant, and long-term.

Psychiatric illness as a result of childbirth

In recent years, psychiatric morbidity postpartum in fathers has come under increasing scrutiny. Studies have looked at couples where the woman has a postpartum depressive disorder that is being treated, and compared them to couples where the woman has no apparent postpartum psychiatric disorder. Spouses of women admitted for their disorder were noted to have a high rate of morbidity—50% (Lovestone & Kumar 1994) and 42% (Harvey & McGrath 1988). The latter study's control group fathers had a 4% morbidity. The diagnosis was most commonly depressive and anxiety disorders, usually of a milder degree than the woman's. Such disorders were associated with discordant marital states and social problems (Harvey & McGrath 1988; Lovestone & Kumar 1994), and with a past psychiatric history and poor relationship with their own father (Lovestone & Kumar 1994).

Another study (Ballard et al 1994) looking at 200 postnatal couples found the prevalence of depression, using the Edinburgh Postnatal Depression Scale (Cox 1983), to be no different to couples with older children. However, mothers had a higher prevalence, and fathers were more likely to be depressed if their wives were.

The father—management issues

The findings of paternal psychiatric morbidity have clear implications for the partners when managing women with postpartum disorders:

1. Partners should always be seen in the initial stages of treatment, and during and on discharge from any in-patient stay.
2. Illness in the partner should always be considered and, if diagnosed, treated appropriately with support and/or therapy and/or medication.
3. Where support and child care is important in the woman's management, it should be discussed with the father, and his ability to assist should not be presumed. *He* may need support and assistance with child care as well as his partner. Night feeds may be difficult for a woman on sedative medication; it may be too great a stress for a depressed father, also trying to keep his job.

Case example

Wendy, 28, was admitted with her infant to a mother-baby unit at 6 weeks postpartum with a major depressive illness. She had previously had counselling but had no other psychiatric history. It was noted that she had been sexually abused as a child by her stepfather and uncle

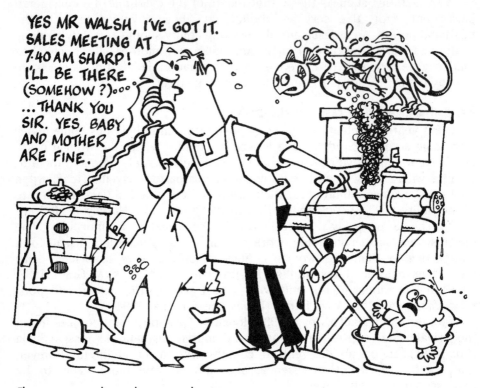

The partner may also need support and assistance

and had a poor relationship with her mother. Wendy and Peter, 32, had been married for 3 years, and had a close and supportive relationship. Peter, an accountant, was bewildered by his wife's marked mood swings and frightened by her suicide threats. He became increasingly depressed after her admission, finding living in an empty house, surrounded by his child's toys, an agonising reminder of dreams that had failed to materialise. He described sleeping difficulties and a decreased appetite. He no longer had Wendy in whom to confide, and felt excluded by her and unable to comprehend her illness. A diagnosis of adjustment disorder with depressed mood was made.

Peter was seen initially by a male psychiatric nurse who runs a weekly fathers' group. In the group setting, Peter was able to express and to understand his anger and his fears. Regular appointments with Wendy's treating doctor were invaluable, keeping Peter in touch with his wife's progress. Later, couple sessions were able to address the impact the arrival of the child and Wendy's illness had had on them, both as a couple and as individuals. These sessions continued after discharge and both parents did well subsequently.

Relationship issues associated with postpartum psychiatric disorder

This can be considered under a number of headings:

Relationship problems as a consequence of the infant or of the maternal depression

The introduction of an infant into a relationship results in a critical period for that relationship. For some couples this period is one of severe crisis, with an increase in resentment and arguments and a decrease in marital satisfaction (Hobbs 1965). The presence of depression in either or both partners will cause added stress. A combination of these factors may contribute to the disintegration of a marriage after the birth of a child. The rate of separation and divorce in psychiatric patients—including psychotic, neurotic and affective disorders, as well as personality disorder and alcoholism—is significantly higher (Dominion 1979). This is even greater where both members have a psychiatric illness (Merikangas 1984).

A study looking at marital adjustment in couples where one was depressed showed significantly worse marital functioning than in other couples (Merikangas et al 1985). Birtchnell and Kennard's study (1983) demonstrated a strong association between a negative marriage score and the diagnosis of depression. Those in the group of patients who had a negative marriage score were more likely to develop psychological morbidity earlier than those with positive scores.

Case example

John, 32, and Carrie, 28, had been married for 5 years. They had 2 girls, Kelly and Brittany, aged 3 years and 6 months, respectively. Both described their marriage prior to the birth of their younger child as good. Their opinions often differed, and arguments were brief and explosive, but were quickly resolved, and balanced by a warm sharing relationship with an active sex life.

With the birth of Brittany, Carrie became increasingly irritable. She felt trapped at home and overwhelmed by her responsibilities. She turned her anger on the older child, whom she hit on a number of occasions. While shopping, she began experiencing panic attacks and became reluctant to leave the house. Her mood was low, worse in the mornings, and she frequently spent most of the day at home in tears.

At night, when John arrived home, he was frustrated by the chaotic situation that greeted him; he frequently chose to stay back late at work, or to go out for a drink with friends to avoid it. When he did arrive home, his tardiness fuelled the already tense and irritable Carrie, who felt angry at having to accept the burden of parenthood without support. Marital fights were frequent and prolonged, and often entailed physical abuse by both parties. Both Carrie and John were highly defensive. John responded to Carrie's verbal tirades and anger at Kelly by becoming increasingly authoritarian and dictatorial with the family. Carrie, who had hated and feared her strict, rigid father, reacted as she had in her adolescence, rebelling in an angry and self-righteous manner.

Carrie was admitted to a mother-baby unit after her treating doctor became concerned about the welfare of her older child. She had been on dothiepin but was concerned about her weight increase and so this was ceased and she was changed to paroxetine. John visited on a number of occasions; on each there were loud arguments. Staff intervened at least once. At this time the staff pointed out how much the depression had affected the relationship, and John was asked how he felt. John admitted to being angry, but agreed that it was only since Brittany's birth that he had felt this way. After being given the opportunity to talk, he was able to remember the positives of their relationship; both he and Carrie agreed to joint sessions.

The couple counselling coincided with an improvement in depressive symptoms in Carrie. These sessions allowed her to vent her anger and frustration in a nonconfrontational manner and she and John were able to unite as parents. The return of 'the couple' within the family was a crucial part of Carrie's recovery. However, even with her depression largely resolved, her relationship with her oldest daughter continued to be difficult. On-going couple work after discharge allowed her to look at the difficulties she had with the child's discipline, with John's input being supportive rather than opposing. They arrived at a solution as a team, and with this unity Kelly's oppositional behaviour quickly settled.

Relationship issues as an aetiological factor in maternal and paternal depression

Studies suggest that rates of admission to psychiatric hospitals are lowest for the married population (Segraves 1980) and that a close confiding relationship has a positive influence on emotional well-being (Brown & Harris 1978).

Other studies have shown the high incidence of negative marital scores in the psychiatrically ill population (Merikangas et al 1985; Birtchnell & Kennard 1983). Studies on postpartum depression have consistently found marital conflict antenatally, particularly with poor sexual relationship, associated with depression developing postpartum (Kendell et al 1981; Kumar & Robson 1984; Dennerstein et al 1989; Robinson & Stewart 1986; Goering et al 1992).

The relationship between marital status, marital discord and psychiatric disability is clearly a complex one, with a number of hypotheses seeking to explain the association (Segraves 1980).

The nature of the marital relationship appears important: marriages with absent or deficient intimacy have a higher association with psychiatric illness (Waring et al 1983).

Segraves (1980) reviews a number of studies which have shown a link with individual psychopathology and later marital difficulties; similarly, high scores of neurosis antenatally in the woman (and psychiatric instability in the spouse) are associated with later depression (Kumar & Robson 1984; Boyce et al 1991; Ballard et al 1994).

While a number of biological, psychological and social factors appear to contribute to the development or recurrence of psychiatric illness postpartum, it seems from these studies that marriages in difficulties prior to the birth of a baby are likely to suffer further. This may then have a further deleterious effect on the psychiatric disorder, or the disorder may further affect the marriage. In this setting both partners will suffer but, interestingly, Feldman et al (1984) found that although symptoms were reported by both partners of maritally distressed couples, wives reported a greater number and intensity of symptoms, particularly agitated depression, somatisation, phobic anxiety and obsessive compulsive neurosis. These are all disorders common in the postpartum period in women; the studies of the husbands report generally less severe symptoms (Harvey & McGrath 1988; Lovestone & Kumar 1994).

It may be that many of the postpartum psychiatric disorders are largely associated with the heightened marital difficulties that arise from having a child, and the inability of the partners to support each other through this transition. Feldman et al (1984) hypothesise that the husbands' responses are less severe because they are less able to express negative emotion, react differently to stress, and because marital harmony may be more central to the woman's psychological well-being.

In clinical practice, couple issues often arise; more often than not, these problems were present to some degree prior to the introduction of children. Fifty per cent of the in-patients of the Mercy Hospital for Women receive couple counselling which continues after discharge. All partners are seen at least once, and some more often.

Absent or no partner

While it appears uncertain if single motherhood in itself is associated with an increased risk of psychiatric illness postpartum, there is a suggestion that admission is more likely to be offered for those presenting, because of often inadequate supports, child care relief and possible risk to the infant. Certainly, where a relationship had broken down during pregnancy or the postpartum period, the woman is presented with extra, major stresses. This may involve grieving, feelings of failure, guilt, regrets and resentment or over-attachment to the child, as well as possible financial burdens.

In caring for single mothers with psychiatric illness, it is important to do the following:

1. Assess the illness in its own right; a depressive illness may be easily glossed over and assumed to be grieving. Severity, symptoms and length of duration of the illness need close scrutiny.
2. Assist, where needed, with social supports offering appropriate social contacts that may provide longstanding support.
3. Offer psychotherapy as appropriate; supportive therapy at least is often an important part of management.
4. Assess possible risk to the child or children; does this woman have a break occasionally, does she have someone to whom to turn when she is ill, or in a crisis?

Case example

Mignon, 19, presented with symptoms of depression at 2 months postpartum. The pregnancy had been unplanned; her parents had pressured the father's child to become engaged, although Mignon had never wished to marry him. At the time of presentation they were living together, but separated 2 weeks later. Mignon's depression, previously attributed to her unhappy relationship, critical parents, marked financial problems, and despair at having to forgo attending university, subsequently worsened. She became suicidal after returning to live with her parents, and was admitted to a mother-baby unit.

After admission, her level of depression was noted as moderately severe and she was commenced on antidepressants. With a lifting in mood, a number of issues arose:

- loss of adolescence, and her grief at having to take on adult responsibility;
- relationship with her parents—she was considered the black sheep and their interaction with her reinforced her adolescence and then criticised it;
- wish to sever ties with the child's father, but feeling guilt at depriving her child;
- guilt at her own rejection of her child.

These issues could only begin to be tackled in hospital, but by establishing confidence in a therapist she was able to start to address them, and to see a direction that had previously been clouded in despair. She did not return to the child's father, although he had regular child access, but she did return to study. Her reliance on her family for child care remains a stumbling block to achieving autonomy, but her gains in other areas of her life have helped her in doing this, and are likely to continue to do so.

The couple—management issues

1. When assessing a psychiatric disorder—in either a woman or a man—where a child is expected, or there is a recent addition, it is crucial to look at the role of psychosocial issues.
2. Whether relationship issues are casual, perpetuating or secondary, if not addressed they are likely to result in prolonged symptomatology. This has implications for the individual, family and child.
3. If a disorder being managed with medication alone fails to respond it is essential to consider other issues.
4. Partners need:
    - to be seen: they can offer a view of the person and the illness from the perspective of someone who has known the patient for a long period of time, and in a different way to the therapist;
    - to be heard: total exclusion from therapy where an infant is involved implies that partners have no role or importance. Couple therapy is

not always indicated, but keeping the partners in contact with what is happening, and allowing them to verbalise their concerns and fears involves them rather than alienates them.

5. Indications for couple therapy:
   - a deterioration in the relationship that does not improve with resolution of the psychiatric disorder;
   - a perceived relationship problem by either partner. Both will need to acknowledge some level of problem to accept therapy, or be able to work in therapy effectively;
   - observed parental pathology that is seen to be affecting the children;
   - observed parental pathology where his or her illness is failing to fully respond to other treatments.

6. It is not easy for couples to change the ways they interact. It takes time and motivation from both parties. This frequently does not exist. But if it is at least brought to the couple's attention at this time, it may be reflected upon and returned to at a later time. Some couples may be motivated for their children, if not for themselves.

Case example – 1

Kelly and Neil, both 27, had been married 2 years when their son Damon was born. Kelly had a history of childhood sexual abuse by an uncle and had been raped at 16. Her father and brother were in gaol on drug charges and her mother had worked as a prostitute. She had a poor relationship with her mother, and Neil's parents rarely spoke to her (although they were accepting of Damon). They lived in a small housing commission flat, and had no social supports (who were acceptable to Kelly, who refused her in-laws' offer).

Kelly was admitted to a mother-baby unit after a second episode of slashing her wrists. She was an in-patient for 12 weeks, with 2 subsequent re-admissions. There were many suicide attempts and she was briefly psychotic. Her diagnosis was a borderline personality disorder with concurrent depression. During this time, Neil was supportive, and caring and understanding to the extreme. Kelly's comments, that he was under the thumb of his mother, and the subversive style exhibited in couple sessions were largely dismissed in view of his overwhelmingly positive front and Kelly's negative self-image.

Kelly was re-admitted, again suicidal, after having a second child. As an in-patient she was difficult, demanding and prone to split staff. A diagnosis of borderline personality disorder was again made. Neil, again, was ever-suffering, sweet and obliging, but quietly critical and undermining.

Three years later, Kelly presented again, pregnant with her third child. In the intervening years, she had left Neil and lost custody of her children on the basis of her psychiatric diagnosis. Since meeting her current partner she had had no psychiatric contact and was on no medication. She presented well, and her partner Dirk confirmed she was, from his perspective, totally normal. He was supportive and affirmative of Kelly.

Kelly's third pregnancy, unlike the first 2, was difficult, with premature labour, foetal distress and her child staying in intensive care for six weeks. Despite this, she remained no more than appropriately anxious. There was no evidence of acting out or of depressed mood; the previous diagnosis of borderline personality disorder was disregarded—this behaviour had *only* been in the setting of depression, and *only* in the setting of an undermining, overly intrusive and critical partner. This was despite a past history that was easily equitable with a borderline personality disorder.

Case example – 2

Cha, 27, and Angela, 26, had known each other for 6 months when she became pregnant. He was a Chinese Vietnamese refugee who had arrived with others of his family in Australia 5 years earlier. He spoke good English and worked as an electrician. Angela, an Anglo-Saxon Australian, had started an interior design course, and worked in a variety of jobs, none of which had lasted longer than a year. Cha's background was of a highly intelligent, close family. Angela had been physically abused as a child, had a poor relationship with both her parents and experienced difficulties in becoming close to anyone.

Following the birth of their child, Angela was unable to cope at home. She moved in with her parents, but found her mother's anxiety heightened her own. She was admitted briefly, in crisis, to a series of mother-baby hospitals before she hit her 10-week-old infant and was referred to a mother-baby unit.

Angela, in hospital, appeared euthymic. She was noted to be very rigid, and coped poorly when her infant acted outside her normal routine. Her de facto visited briefly, but avoided staff. She denied any relationship issues.

On the first leave at home, Angela rang the unit 1 hour after arriving at home, in the middle of a panic attack. Her de facto had taken her to 'her' home and left for the night to stay with his family. Angela had been unable to connect his repeated absences, his affiliation with his own family, and their essentially separate residences with her own symptoms. She had coped with her earlier emotional traumas by separating herself emotionally from reality. The result was that she had little insight into her current stressors and how to deal with them.

Angela's psychopathology was long-standing; she needed long-term individual work to come to terms with her own issues. At the same time, however, the involvement of Cha was essential—initially for the safety and care of their child, and then to look at whether their relationship as a couple was viable. They came from vastly different backgrounds, culturally and emotionally. Although in the short term

Cha was able to offer Kelly support, her long-term conflicts were too demanding for him to deal with. Couple work did not succeed in maintaining their relationship—which at best had only ever been tentative—but it did help ensure the infant's safety, and gave Angela a far better male model to which to refer in subsequent therapy than her father had previously been.

Case example – 3

Caroline, 40, had been married to Joshua, 30, for 2 years. Their infant twins were 3 months old when she was referred to a psychiatrist. Joshua had been in personal therapy for 5 years; Caroline had 'no idea' why. She had met him at a disco, and married him 3 months later. She described a series of brief relationships, and a fear of the impending '40' and of her possible inability to have children. She had fallen pregnant immediately, but had had a miscarriage. Her subsequent pregnancy was arduous and had required her to give up work because of pre-eclampsia. Joshua was studying at this time, and the 4-times-a-week psychotherapy debt continued to rise.

Joshua attended an appointment with Caroline's psychiatrist reluctantly. He felt that the whole problem was Caroline's. He said that after the birth of the twins he had (reluctantly) returned to work. They were living with her parents for financial reasons; he argued frequently with her mother and 'despised' her father. He refused to discuss much of why he was in therapy, but spoke of his (female) therapist in terms of a mother figure, and admitted he considered Caroline in a similar way. Caroline, rather than being surprised or repulsed, accepted this, but felt that the arrival of 2 'real' infants meant that she now had only limited time and capacity to mother her husband. Over several joint sessions, rather than electing to alter this relationship substantially, she chose to continue to 'mother' all 3, and he accepted his children in terms of sibling rivals. The longevity of this relationship, however, has to be questioned.

CHAPTER 6

Beyond the couple

Cultural issues

Attitudes to motherhood, fatherhood and child rearing differ widely between Western and other cultures. Some research has suggested that postpartum depression is not as common in other cultures and that the higher incidence of postpartum depression in Western cultures is a result of a lack of systemised support and assistance, and lack of recognition of status (Stern & Kruckman 1983).

In a review, Cox (1988) describes a variety of rituals in societies in China, Jamaica and India where, following childbirth, the woman receives considerable extra support and attention.

Macintyre (1992) describes the attitude to childbirth in Papua New Guinea as supportive, well educated (on the process of pregnancy and birth) and that any lowered mood is treated pragmatically and in context. The role of child rearer is highly valued—the emphasis is on rearing, rather than producing. As well, in non-Western cultures, it is much more likely that there are enforced rituals, mandatory rest and assistance. Cox (1988) suggests that this enhances self-esteem, supports the marital relationship and enforces status.

In Western cultures, the emphasis on and value given to child rearing is quite different. Many women feel caught between the old and new with unsupportive, 'traditional' partners, and little society support or sense of value for their contribution. The dilemma of work versus child rearing is very real for some women, who may be disappointed at their lack of enjoyment of something that was often planned and wanted, and guilty at wanting to and/or returning to an old lifestyle at work, where their role is more valued. For others, due to the costs of child care, and the inadequate availability of part-time work, there is no choice—and they remain torn between disappointment and guilt, often angry at their partner, who has escaped the dilemma. I saw one woman, previously a successful manager, now full-time at home, who told me that one of her biggest fears was being asked that innocuous cliché question—'And what do you do?'.

For other women living in a Western country, but whose heritage is non-Western, there may be cultural issues pertinent to presentation postpartum with psychiatric illness.

Their cultural expectations may not be met, or may be opposed by Western health professionals and services not aware of these expectations, during pregnancy or the postpartum. Insensitivity to privacy and to a dress code, or instructions of an early return to 'normal' physical duties where cultures advocate long rest periods, can produce misunderstandings, guilt and fear—and noncompliance.

In some Asian cultures there are very specific rituals related to childbirth that are crucial to physical and mental well-being. A spirituality may be associated with childbirth that is quite different to that experienced (or experienced but disregarded) in Western cultures. Rice et al (1994) reported a case of a Hmong woman whose health had deteriorated postpartum. The woman attributed this to the loss of her soul during a Caesarean section. Her health returned to normal following a culturally sensitive intervention.

Relatives may also be unable to meet expectations of support and care, due to their 'Westernisation', separation by long distance, work commitments, or lack of awareness where a cross-cultural marriage has occurred.

These women may have the added stress of trauma from their own backgrounds, in the case of refugees for instance, and may be separated from or have lost relatives who would normally be caring for them. Some women experience much suffering, the birth of a child highlighting how much they miss their own family. For those who still have family alive, reuniting may be too costly—either financially or politically—or even if possible, may only be temporary.

Women from some cultures arriving in Australia may experience a 'downgrading' professionally and socially, and with the move to Australia lose the facility to be supported by servants. Many Malaysian professional women, for instance, would be expected to do minimal housework or child care in their home country; the reality of motherhood in Australia for professional women is combining both with their paid job.

For many recent immigrants, language may be a problem, adding to isolation. Local services may be inadequate or inappropriate; these women may also be unaware of them.

Cultural issues—management issues

1. In areas in Australia of high immigration, cultural awareness is generally increasing, as are appropriate services. If treating someone from a culture you know little about, try to find out about the culture's attitudes to pregnancy, childbirth and child rearing, and inquire about the details of immigration—did the woman want to come, or was she forced to (either by circumstances or her partner)? Most importantly, what family does she have available, and are they appropriate as supports?
2. Where English is not spoken, or not spoken well, an independent interpreter may be a valuable source of cultural information, and be less

biased and more accurate than family members. Psychiatric symptoms may present differently—ask the interpreter how the woman appears to him or her, and how culturally appropriate her comments are.

3. In Western society, mental illness is stigmatised. In many European and Asian cultures this stigma is extreme. In these cultures, secrecy may be crucial, keeping the illness hidden even from other family members. In some cases, having a sibling with a mental illness will affect the marriageability of the well sibling. The use of an interpreter, particularly where the community is small, may be feared; it is essential that confidentiality is maintained and that the woman and her family are reassured of this.

4. Where possible, find culturally appropriate supports.

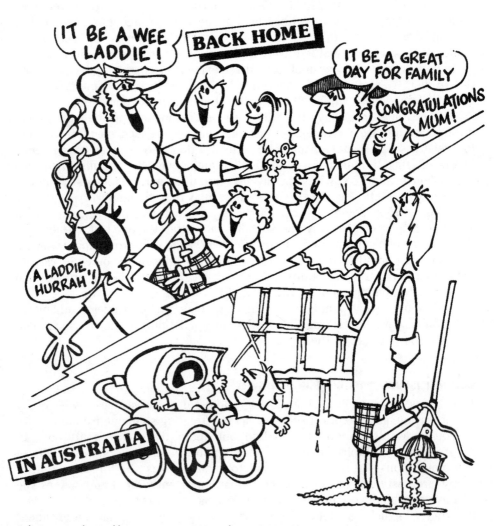

Relatives may be unable to meet expectations due to separation

5. When you are seeing someone from a culture of which you know little, it can be difficult to keep the balance of respect and professional inquiry; beware of stereotypes (although don't necessarily ignore them altogether), and be guided by the woman's responses.

Case example – 1

Chu, a 28-year-old Vietnamese woman, was admitted from a hostel for refugees where the hostel workers had become increasingly concerned about her detachment from her 2-month-old daughter, Rose. Chu had been in Australia for 2 years, following an arranged marriage to a Vietnamese-born Australian citizen. In Vietnam, she had grown up in a well-educated, wealthy family, but her father had been arrested on political grounds and later died while imprisoned. Her family had subsequently lost their wealth and influence and saw the marriage as a way out for their daughter.

Chu's husband had misrepresented himself to her family. In her new country, where she spoke only basic English, she had lived with her in-laws and was used as a maid. Her husband's uncle had made frequent advances to her, and when she had become pregnant her husband had thrown her out of the house, installed his lover and claimed that the child was not his.

Chu, a moral and respectful person, had been devastated. She was totally isolated from her family and friends, and limited by her lack of language skills. She felt unable to return home because of 'loss of face', fearing that her family would believe her husband's claims that she was bearing an illegitimate child, and that 'whoring behaviour' of which she had been accused, would ostracise her in her home country. As a result, she felt life was not worth living, and had had difficulties bonding to her child, who in some ways she felt was responsible for her predicament.

Chu unfolded much of this story over time, tempering trust with caution. Interestingly, she was more willing to express herself in English—fearful that the interpreter (also Vietnamese), might slander her in the Vietnamese community. Although this in no way reflects the interpreter's professionalism, it shows the tight-knit nature of small ethnic communities.

In this case, nurturing, supportive and uncritical care was essential; a Vietnamese counsellor (who assured Chu of confidentiality) was also an important component of the management plan. The most important part, however, was convincing her family of origin that the child was indeed her husband's; fortunately, their level of medical knowledge meant that DNA testing was acceptable proof.

Case example – 2

Ivan, 30, and Domenica, 23, presented when Domenica was 28 weeks pregnant with their second child. After the birth of their son, now 2,

Domenica had been depressed for 6 months, but had received no treatment. The couple stated that they were keen 'not to have a recurrence' of the experience.

Ivan and Domenica had been married for 4 years. Domenica had been born in southern Italy but raised in Australia since the age of 3 months. Ivan was born in Australia of Yugoslav parents. Domenica had always had a difficult relationship with her father, whom she saw as domineering and rigid; this was amplified by her marriage, as her father was unaccepting and critical of Ivan, whose cultural background he regarded as inferior.

Domenica connected her depression following her son's birth with the argument that had ensued over the child's name (according to the southern Italian tradition, this should have been the name of the paternal grandfather; Domenica's father insisted that it should be his) and over the godparents (from Ivan's family, not Domenica's). This had resulted in Ivan and Domenica refusing to speak to her father; Domenica had been further traumatised by her mother turning against her daughter in support of her husband.

Domenica fantasised that this new child would reunite the family; therapy focused on her acceptance of her mother's position, which had always been to follow her husband, and that this did not necessarily reflect on Domenica as a person, nor on her mother's love for her. In the second step, a move from placing the wishes of their parents paramount towards a greater care for their own family was essential for them to escape the boundaries and use their own potentials within the relationship, for themselves and for their children.

Life events and social support

Many researchers have linked episodes of psychiatric illness to excessively stressful life events and to inadequate social supports. It has been suggested that social support may be protective; other researchers have suggested that inadequate support may produce symptomatology (Aneshensel & Stone 1982). Social support is also seen to have an important role in recovery; Breier and Strauss (1984) detail how helpful such support can be for psychotic patients in returning to reality and in coming to terms with their illness.

Studies of postpartum disorders have generally reported that women who develop postpartum depression also have a higher incidence of stressful life events, and that this appears particularly important if combined with a poor marital relationship (Paykel et al 1980; O'Hara 1986), although it has been suggested that this is a perception affecting depression (Henderson et al 1991). Women who experienced higher stress tended to have longer lasting emotional problems (Gordon et al 1965), and emotional support has been linked to self-esteem and to parenting attitudes (Rogosch et al 1992).

Psychiatric illness in itself brings with it social and interpersonal adjustment difficulties. Although this improves with the symptoms, it may be slower to do so, and may not resolve completely (Paykel & Weissman 1973).

Clinically, there are a number of particularly stressful life events that are common. Childbirth in itself is a physical and social stress with effects, as discussed in other chapters, on the relationship between partners and the families of origin. It also entails a role change for the women. Ceasing paid employment may be temporary or permanent—the choice can be stressful, but so can the change in the financial situation. Women who have previously been independent may find it difficult to adapt to asking their husband for money; the changes financially and through the advent of the baby may alter their lifestyle considerably with less (or no) entertaining, spontaneous weekends away or evenings out together.

When pregnancy is confirmed, it is a common time for reassessing living arrangements; renovations or moves begun at this time are all too often coming to fruition just at the time of delivery. The new mother returns home to pack years of accumulated belongings, or else to contend with protecting the infant's oxygen and oral intake from layers of plaster dust. Moving may mean isolation from a familiar environment and social network. International relocation—often avoided until after the baby is born, but only by weeks or months—brings a particular isolation which can act to bring the family unit closer together, but often represents a major challenge to the new mother. Unlike her husband, who has a ready-made social network through work, a network must be actively sought.

For those couples who decide not to move, the attitude to the family home and surrounding area can change. What was suitable for a working couple who spent little time at home may not be as desirable for a mother unable to get out often. Accessibility of family, friends and facilities such as the maternal-child health nurse, becomes crucial.

A number of other stresses are also likely to confront new couples: christenings, Christmas or family get-togethers may present women with a dilemma—they may feel they must prepare a magnificent spread, but they are in fact tired and unenthusiastic about attending, let alone hosting, such an event.

Women postpartum are also likely to be particularly sensitive to life events such as murders, war and famine, particularly where children are involved. For those women already barely coping, graphic media coverage can be extremely stressful, and for those women with intrusive, obsessional thoughts, common in depression at this time, such reports can precipitate thoughts of 'what if I were to do that…'.

Life events and social support—management issues

By the time these women present, the stresses are usually already operating, and the social networks are perceived as inadequate; however, the clinician can assist by:

1. assessing the current role of any stressors. Look at what can be done to minimise their effects. Can moving, christenings or family events be postponed, or can someone else be enlisted to help? The woman herself will often say that there is no one, but partners or other family members may be able to assess the situation from a broader and more realistic perspective. If renovations are in progress, would it be possible to live elsewhere temporarily (as long as this wouldn't create a greater problem either financially or through the stress of living with in-laws)?
2. assessing social supports and encouraging development or improvement. This may need to involve the partner: looking at the social changes in their relationship, the possibility of some evenings out, and the availability of babysitters. It is not uncommon for the male partner to be more enthusiastic about this than the new mother, but this is an important part of the pendulum which, having swung from couple to mother and infant, needs to be re-balanced between the 2. Other networks are important. For mothers who have previously worked full-time and who may have had little to do with other mothers and young children, new mothers' groups (run by maternal-child health nurses) can be an important social and educational support. Some areas also have specific groups, such as for young mothers, or for particular ethnic groups. Involvement in other activities such as yoga, craft or sport can be beneficial in themselves, as well as be a means of increasing networks.

Case example – 1

Heather, 35, became pregnant while having an affair. Her husband was sterile and the affair was, in part, a result of Heather's unconscious desire to have children. Her husband divorced her and she married the father of the child. Her own parents had separated when she had been a child and her mother had suffered from chronic depression. Heather had worked in a managerial role in a large department store and had enjoyed a successful career until the birth of her child.

Heather became suicidally depressed and required an in-patient admission. Her acute symptoms settled with medication, but her mood remained low, she felt inadequate as a mother and was despairing of the future. She was observed to be loving and caring of her infant but was at times overwhelmed with the responsibility. In couple counselling it quickly became evident that Heather had little in common with her new husband, Michael.

After discharge, the family moved to the outskirts of the city at Michael's insistence, for 'the health of their child'. As there was only one car, which he took to work, and no public transport, this meant that Heather was isolated.

Heather became pregnant again while still mildly depressed and on medication, when her elder child was 1 year old. She ceased taking the antidepressant immediately, for fear of its effect on her unborn child. Her condition deteriorated, and she was admitted once during the pregnancy, and immediately postpartum. The depression continued through the pregnancy and for many months postpartum it appeared resistant to all forms of therapy. Michael refused to be involved.

With Heather's youngest now aged 2 years, she continued in a difficult marriage, had significant depressive symptoms and experienced feelings of guilt, despair and inadequacy. Her husband's job then forced a move to the country, where she was referred for long-term therapy, but where few supports were available.

Heather's own mental health, that of her children and the viability of the family unit long term, must be questioned. Her mother's history of chronic depression seemed set to repeat itself; this had been associated with parental divorce, which all too likely may also be repeated.

An intelligent woman, Heather had been overwhelmed by her life circumstances, and was unable to take on responsibilities. Individual therapy could help her look at her own feelings of powerlessness and the pull of repeating patterns. Ideally, this would have occurred prior to having children. Had Michael been willing, couple therapy might have been able to address the many marital problems. The case highlights, all too clearly, how often the therapist is unable to intervene and how therapy can be sabotaged. The management of Heather's illness was limited by her isolation; her experience of depression was significantly worsened by feeling trapped, and by lack of access to a peer group that might have assisted her self-esteem and helped her to hold on to that part of her which had previously contributed to her success as a manager.

Case example – 2

Toni, 26, had an unplanned pregnancy after a prior termination. Her de facto, Will, left her when she was 3 months pregnant after a violent argument in which her arm had been broken. There was a reconciliation a month prior to their son's birth; they moved interstate at this time to get away from her mother, whom Will saw as a negative influence.

Toni delivered in a hospital with which she was unfamiliar; the labour was prolonged, the infant became distressed and was delivered by forceps with a third-degree tear to the mother. She required several hospitalisations due to retained placental products and infective complications, including mastitis.

Despite this horrendous introduction to motherhood, Toni coped remarkably well; she related later that the hospitalisations had in fact created a temporary network—it was only after her final discharge that she felt overwhelmingly alone. Pain, with which she had previously dealt without analgesics, worsened and required frequent trips to casualty for pethidine injections.

Toni was finally referred to a psychiatrist for an assessment by protective services, following their involvement after another violent argument with Will, in which Toni had threatened to harm her child, feeling overwhelmed by her responsibilities and angry at how unaffected Will had been in comparison. At the initial presentation she was angry rather than depressed, but with clear evidence of a deterioration in her capacity to cope with day-to-day life, she revealed over a number of weeks a pattern of reacting to stress by becoming angry that could be traced back to adolescence. Her elderly parents had been rigid disciplinarians, which had induced her to rebel. She had been, and had remained, angry at them.

Without social supports, and with a number of severe physical stresses, Toni put increasing reliance on an already shaky relationship; the final breaking point came when Will left her, and Toni became suicidal.

Management was needed to first address relationship issues, improving Toni's self-esteem and helping Toni decide whether or not to return to her home town. Before she was able to make this decision, she had to come to terms with the fact that the relationship was over, and with the prospect of being a single mother. Returning home was not a solution; her relationship with her mother was difficult, and her peers did not have children. Linking in to a new mothers' group, family aid and child care workers visiting at home, as well as individual therapy, were part of a long-term management plan.

In each of these cases, stresses were multiple, and were connected with other relevant factors, both past and present. While not all cases are as complex, such stories are not unusual. These complexities, the high level of life events and marital and family of origin issues, predispose women to develop psychiatric illness—particularly postpartum when the stress of child care is constant and, for many, inescapable.

CHAPTER 7

The mother–infant relationship

The mother–infant bond

The relationship between mother and child, that begins at conception and is nurtured throughout pregnancy, finally becomes very real at birth. Klaus and Kennell (1975) proposed that women were hormonally sensitised at birth to 'bond' with their infant, a notion that has become popular, although it does not always occur. Bowlby (1969) expanded this notion in his attachment theory, highlighting the importance for later development of a secure attachment by an infant to a caregiver in the first year of life. Hopkins (1990) summarises this as pre-programmed behaviour with an evolutionary basis.

The mother, in synchrony with her child, learns the soothing nature of her body and the particular tones of her voice to which the child responds. Mothers who are secure in themselves enable babies to form a secure attachment through which they learn to understand themselves and their environment.

Ainsworth (1975), in looking at infant–mother attachment, found that not all mothers and infants appeared to form this secure attachment. By looking at maternal behaviours and infant responses, she found two other types of attachment—avoidant and ambivalent. These observations on the Ainsworth Strange Situation test (1971) can also be observed in the home environment: this test essentially looks at the infant's reaction to separation from its mother, and to her return. Secure attachments are associated with happier, co-operative babies, where mothers respond sensitively and appropriately. Avoidant attachments are associated with mothers who appear uncomfortable with physical and emotional closeness, and infants who appear, as a result, to become isolated and self-contained. Ambivalent attachments form where the mother is insecure and erratic and responds to the baby more in response to her own needs; the infant is frustrated and angry at the inconsistency.

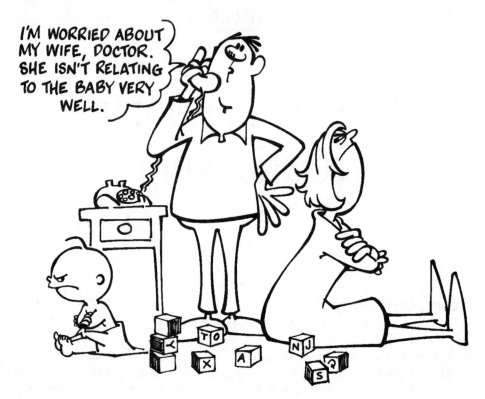

Not all mothers and infants appear to form a secure attachment

The mother

Many factors contribute to the attachment of the mother to her infant. In the mother these include a biological influence as well as psychosocial factors, both in the immediate setting as well as from the past. Cohler et al's study (1980) of parenting attitudes and child development noted that pregnancy and birth complications adversely affected such attitudes, in both mentally ill and well women. They also concluded that these attitudes, as a reflection of the mother's personality, were associated with a child's impaired cognitive development and with negative maternal behaviour.

Maternal attitudes and the ability to form a secure attachment are likely to depend on a number of factors. A background of emotional deprivation and/or physical/sexual abuse, an inadequate early attachment or later problems in the relationship with the woman's own mother, or an inadequate or absent role model are factors likely to influence the new mother's attitudes and confidence.

Current psychopathology is likely to contribute to a lowering of the mother's self-esteem, confidence, concentration and capacity to relate to a dependent infant sensitively and appropriately. A past history of a poor relationship with her own mother from infancy or childhood, also more likely in women with a psychiatric history, will leave the woman without a role model and with a heightened anxiety not to repeat her mother's mistakes. Lack of support, particularly in the marital relationship, will further impair the capacity to consistently and confidently provide a secure emotional environment.

The infant

Many clinicians, and indeed mothers, underestimate the contributions made by the baby to the relationship. While many are quick to label a baby 'difficult' or 'temperamental', there is less understanding of the infant's capacity for cognition and response. Murray (1989) reviewed the increasingly refined experiments looking at infants (and indeed the foetus) which demonstrate a high degree of emotional synchrony. Other studies have shown facial expressions and responses to adult communications, and the ability to distinguish the mother's face in babies as young as 6 weeks.

While the infant may indeed be 'pre-programmed' to attach, there appears to be a capacity to respond—and therefore a variety of responses to a variety of stimuli—which suggests that the development will be sensitive to the particular stimuli (and mother) to which it is exposed.

Much of the infant's early awareness is watching its mother's face and listening to her voice. The child is dependent on its mother to be 'contained' (Bion 1962) physically and emotionally, that is, provided with a supportive, nurturing and safe environment, and from this experience memories are being formed. The infant relies on its mother, but has the capacity to learn from experience, and experiences vary. Development is reliant on genetics, and complex factors associated with the responsiveness of both the infant and its parent(s).

Infants of mothers with a psychiatric illness are at an increased risk of forming an insecure attachment.

The association between psychiatric disorders in parents and behavioural disturbances in children: the mechanisms

The link between psychiatric illness in parents and disturbances in their offspring has been known for many years (Cox et al 1987). Quinton and Rutter proposed the mechanisms of the association could be:

1. genetic;
2. direct impact of the parental disorder;
3. indirect effects of the parental disorder;
4. ill effects of the factors associated with the disorder.

In practice, it is hard to establish which, if any, is the primary aetiology. Psychiatric illness will often produce an altered relationship, impaired parenting, and separations via hospitalisation and family disruption. Many studies have looked at these issues; most concluded that there was an association of more than one aspect in the parental illness with childhood disturbance.

Depression

A number of studies in recent years have focused on the outcome of the children of women who have been depressed following childbirth. The premise of many of these studies is that the relationship of depressed mothers and their children is impaired, and that this may have long-term consequences. Observations include that these relationships have been characterised by rejection, anxiety, over-protection and guilt (Uddenberg 1974), that depressed mothers are likely to be less responsive and less able to sustain social interaction and that mothers are more restricted in how they structure family life and in the guidance of children (Cox et al 1987).

My own observation of depressed mothers and their infants under 12 months is that the mothers tend to fall into 1 of 2 groups:

1. those who are warm and loving but who are low in self-esteem, and feel guilty at their perceived inadequacy as a mother, and have difficulty allowing others to assist in child care. They set unrealistic agendas for themselves, and are often rigid in their expectations of self and child;
2. those who have difficulties connecting with their infant. They are usually aware that they have not 'bonded' in some way with their child, but their own defences against intimacy prevent them opening up to their child, as it would render them too vulnerable. They are often competent practically as mothers, but appear clinical.

The impairment of relationship between depressed mothers and their children has been largely substantiated by long-term studies on children up to 4½ years, which have linked maternal depression to childhood behavioural problems and cognitive impairment.

Depressed mothers generally rated their children's behaviour as difficult (Brody & Forehand 1986; Caplan et al 1989; Lee & Gotlib 1989). Kelly (1976) suggested that the woman's depression and her response to her infant may be affected by her infant's temperament, while other authors have suggested that the depressed woman's perceptions of difficulty is increased (Hopkins et al 1984). In Lee and Gotlib's study (1989), the researchers also considered the children to be difficult.

There is less agreement about the association between later childhood behavioural and cognitive impairment and the timing of the depression. Janson (1993) found an association with antenatal but not postnatal depression or depression at 3 years after the birth. Wrate et al (1985) found an association with brief depression but not prolonged, Coghill et al (1986) with depression in the first year, and Uddenberg and Englesson (1978) with prolonged, recurrent depression. Caplan et al (1989) found no link with postnatal depression, but did find other associated factors which correlated with childhood difficulties.

Other factors—marital disharmony and paternal psychiatric history—were found to be significant in both Caplan et al's study (1989) and Coghill et al's study (1986). In each of these studies, children with these factors present scored significantly lower on the McCarthy scale of cognitive ability.

While there are some differences between these studies, all essentially link maternal depression and/or associated marital problems and paternal psychiatric illness (more likely to be present—see Chapter 5) with childhood difficulties.

Of particular concern is that it may only require a disorder of brief duration (Wrate et al 1985) to set into motion an impairment in the mother-infant relationship from which it may not recover. The negative, rejecting relationship observed by Uddenberg and Englesson (1978) in more women with more prolonged depressive episodes may represent another end of the same scale.

Given that we also know that a family history of depression, and an impaired parental relationship, predisposes women to postpartum depression, the seed is being set in infancy for a recurring pattern.

Depression—management issues

In the management of any woman with postpartum depression, the infant is an integral part of the illness and its management.

1. Always see the mother with her baby.
2. Listen to how she speaks about the child. Be alert to feelings of anxiety, inadequacy and anger. Allow the woman to vent these feelings.
3. It is all right to give feedback. Sometimes, being told that it is normal to feel frustrated and despairing if a baby will not settle can be reassuring.
4. Although these women are not easily reassured, reality testing is important. Many have constructed a very unrealistic, perfect reality for themselves. Challenge it, and help them to challenge it also. Ask them to tell you, or write down, what their concept of a good mother is, and then go through each item with them.

   For instance, why does a good mother have to wash the floors every day? What is the worst that will happen if she doesn't? How realistic is that? How can a mother ever know exactly why her child is crying *every* time?
5. Watch, where possible, the woman with her infant. Look at how she responds (or doesn't respond) to cues; point out where the baby does seem to be responding to its mother or the environment.
6. In de-emphasising the importance of many of the rules—often involving practical issues—that the woman has constructed, promote the importance of what the woman is able to do well and what she can do that is 'good mothering', that is, the time spent with her child. Many of these mothers do not appreciate the interactive and receptive ability of their young infants.

   It is important that such play and interaction not be destructive. Depressed women can be over-involved and attempt to over-stimulate the infant in response to their guilt. Suggest the mother watch her infant, and be guided by it. Baby massage is a good way of helping both the over-involved mother and the detached mother become more aware of their infant.

7. Where there is sustained impairment in the interaction, even after the mother's depression has lifted or is lifting, or where the depression is slow to lift, a more formal therapy for the mother and infant is recommended, preferably with a psychologist or psychiatrist specialising in this area. Some centres are able to offer group or individual mother-infant work. In view of the long-term research findings, such referrals should not be delayed.

Case example – 1

Katrina, 31, a married occupational therapist, was admitted at 6 weeks postpartum with symptoms of depression since immediately after the birth of her daughter, Maddison. She became increasingly withdrawn and was noted to be mechanical with her child. She described feeling 'peculiar' at the birth, and said that although she knew Maddison was her child, she felt no connection. She said that she could observe that the infant was well formed, and even attractive, but that she felt nothing. Over several weeks as an in-patient, although her mood lifted a little, she remained depressed and related poorly to Maddison. She was reluctant to take the child to groups with her, and reacted with obvious relief whenever a nurse offered to care for Maddison.

Katrina had a history of marked emotional deprivation. Her parents had separated when she was 3 and, although officially in the care of her mother, she spent months at a time in foster care, separated from her only sister and with no knowledge of her father's whereabouts. Her mother had had frequent psychiatric hospitalisations associated with depression and suicide attempts. At 12, she was reunited with her father and a stepmother, but after a traumatic year she was returned to foster care. At 15, while with her mother, they argued and her mother committed suicide; Katrina found the body. As a result, Katrina was left feeling responsible, that she had been rejected by her father, and that her mother had thought her such a bad person that she had killed herself rather than remain with Katrina.

Throughout Katrina's life, particularly following her mother's suicide, she put up barriers to closeness. To get close was to be vulnerable; rejection was too great a pain for her to bear. Her husband Greg was described as supportive, but had little understanding of the degree of emotional turmoil that existed just below the surface. Their relationship had largely survived because his night shifts ensured they had little time together.

Faced with an infant, Katrina's own raw vulnerability was mirrored and she withdrew in terror. Holding the infant reminded her of how she had wanted to be held; such memories were terrifying, a reliving of an infancy and childhood without security.

In the ward setting, encouragement of the development of the relationship between Katrina and Maddison could proceed only slowly. Baby massage terrified Katrina; she saw the naked child as vulnerable and exposed. Her method of dealing with baths and nappy changes was to do so quickly and methodically; baby massage asked her to maintain attention on the child, which she was unable to do. The first step then was to have very brief sessions with a nurse present, and Katrina and the nurse would observe Maddison. The nurse would occasionally draw attention to what developmental tasks Maddison had achieved, and invite Katrina to observe these, and in particular how Maddison responded and interacted with her mother. Katrina seemed surprised that the nurse felt that Maddison recognised her as her mother, but started believing this over a number of sessions.

Katrina's subsequent management is long-term. Unfortunately, she felt unable to attend a mother-infant therapist, and it was left to the individual therapist to reintroduce this concept after Katrina worked through her own issues. In the meantime, Maddison was placed in a full-time crèche. This will possibly provide Maddison with some stimulation, but bypasses the mother–infant relationship. The reality, however, is that for some women, particularly those from deprived and abusive backgrounds, until the individual issues are resolved, the involvement of the infant is not possible. The individual therapist in such a situation must keep the infant in mind—just as surely as Katrina was trying to keep Maddison out of hers—so that therapy can progress to include the relationship with the child.

Case example – 2

Arlene, 36, was a deputy headmistress who, with her husband Ian, 48, also a teacher, had decided not to have children. An unplanned pregnancy was greeted with shock but, due to a religious background, a termination was not an option. The pregnancy meant a promotion had to be declined, and a new city flat they had just moved into was sold in favour of a suburban house.

Labour was prolonged and traumatic. Arlene became severely depressed with vegetative symptoms and suicidal thoughts. Her child, Darcy, was born with talipes, which Arlene regarded as God's punishment for not wanting the child. Arlene was placed under 24-hour observation. She was able to do little for Darcy, referring to her as 'the baby'. There was no eye contact and little spontaneity in her child care. She was relieved to have Darcy cared for, and on several occasions requested she be sent to her mother's or sister's.

Ian appeared bewildered by fatherhood, but was openly supportive and caring of his wife. Arlene's mother was at times intrusive but also supportive. Arlene described a difficult relationship as a teenager with her devoutly religious mother but felt that they had become closer in recent years. Her father had a history of alcoholism and had physically abused his wife, but Arlene and her siblings had been protected from this.

After 2 weeks on high doses of antidepressants, Arlene's mood began to lift steadily. Four weeks after admission, she was euthymic and although apprehensive about how she would adjust to being at home with an infant, was able to discuss this and make appropriate plans. Most interestingly, her relationship with Darcy changed dramatically. The infant was described as wanted, and although she was unplanned, she would change nothing. Arlene became warm and spontaneous, with good eye contact, and was able to respond appropriately to Darcy's cues. The talipes became a minor nuisance rather than an issue.

It is important to remember that not all depressed women will have long-term problems in their relationship with their infant. Although Arlene's background was perhaps not perfect, it appears to have provided her with a sense of self and a 'good enough' role model. The brevity of this depressive episode, although severe, may also have limited any guilt and feelings of inadequacy she had felt as a mother.

Psychotic disorders

Studies of families of people with psychotic disorders, essentially schizophrenia and bipolar disorder, have documented the high risk of such disorders developing in offspring. This risk exists even where the child of psychotic parents is raised by another family, suggesting a strong genetic predisposition.

Parnas and Jorgensen (1987) looked at 175 offspring of 129 psychotic mothers (Copenhagen project) at a mean age of 25 years: 15 (9%) had developed schizophrenia, 29 a schizotypal personality disorder (17%) and 42 (24%) a paranoid personality. This compared to 1%, 1% and 4.5%, respectively, of the control group. The authors associated maternal early onset, non-paranoid schizophrenia and antisocial personality traits, as well as an impaired parent–child relationship, parental absence and institutional rearing, with later development of schizophrenia.

There was also a higher incidence of pregnancy and birth complications. The authors concluded that these children had a genetic predisposition, but that this was mediated by environmental factors. Emery et al (1982), however, found marital discord not to be a mediating factor in schizophrenia.

Studies comparing mothering in women with psychotic disorders to well women have found a number of significant differences. Cohler et al (1980) studied 48 women, two-thirds of whom had a schizophrenic illness and one-third a bipolar disorder, and their children at ages 3 to 5 years. They found that these women, compared to normal controls, did not value reciprocal communication and had difficulties distinguishing their own needs from that of their children. These attitudes were associated with retardation of their children's cognitive development. In this study, schizophrenic mothers were withdrawn and emotionally uninvolved with their children. A number of researchers concluded that it is the *severity* and *chronicity* of the disorder that is most related to childhood outcome (Sameroff et al 1982; Rogosch et al 1992).

Psychotic disorders—management issues

Major issues that need to be considered:
1. capacity to care for the infant;
2. need for protective services;
3. use of long-term community services to address parental issues, for instance, services such as family and parenting education;
4. long-term community services to address the physical and emotional development of the child, particularly where:
   - both parents have a psychiatric disorder;
   - mother is noncompliant and/or insightless;
   - there is minimal or no family supports and/or backup;
   - marital discord exists.

Case example – 1

Lucy, a 29-year-old Chinese woman, presented at 27 weeks pregnant, requesting a termination. She spoke good English, having lived in Australia for 5 years. Two months prior she had separated from her husband and was living alone. Neighbours had noticed peculiar behaviour (for instance, standing outside in one spot for long periods of time, wearing her night attire to the shops). Her flat was unkempt, with a fridge full of half-eaten food, some mouldy. She denied any hallucinations and there was no apparent thought disorder. Although reluctant to discuss it, she had paranoid fears that her husband had been harmed, and had rung the police on a number of occasions.

Lucy had had two previous psychiatric admissions for brief psychotic disorders. In the intervening time there had been psycho-social deterioration, prompting the separation from her husband. She had no family or friends.

The most likely diagnosis was schizophrenia.

The specific management concerns were her insightlessness, and lack of supports. In particular, she also had little concept of the infant inside her—she alternated between asking blandly for a termination, and then declaring warmly how much she loved the child. Such ambivalence needed close assessment: if this continued to be present after the birth of the child, her capacity to consistently care for the infant would be severely impaired. Both the physical and emotional development of the child could be affected.

The time remaining in the pregnancy was used to put supports in place, with a child care assessment and mental state examination mandatory before her discharge from hospital.

Case example – 2

Tania, a 17-year-old single woman, was admitted 4 months after her daughter Monique was born. Tania had paranoid delusions, fearing that her daughter was going to be kidnapped and that she herself was on an ASIO 'hit list'. She had no past psychiatric history, but had a history of sexual abuse by an uncle, and had left school at an early age. She had had several jobs of only weeks' or months' duration.

Tania's parents had separated when she was 3. She was an only child who had since lived with her mother. Her mother, Kaye, had had a history of schizophrenia since Tania's birth, and this had been untreated. Kaye presented well, but at an interview appeared mildly thought-disordered, and with an extensive delusional system, also featuring ASIO.

Tania described a disturbed childhood where she had had to fend for herself from a young age, at times also for, or against, her mother. Even when recovered from this episode, her thinking was at times magical and bordering on delusional. It is tempting to speculate that the environment in which she was raised influenced this.

Tania's relationship with Monique was caring and warm. In the acute phase, however, the delusion relating to Monique being poisoned meant that solids were ceased. When the acute phase settled, although her mothering skills were good, there was concern about her ability to be consistent, given that her mental state still fluctuated. Her ability to distinguish reality from delusions remained an issue, particularly as she worked through issues relating to her own childhood sexual abuse. The long-term effect on Monique is unknown. The potential for a repeating pattern is worrying.

Other psychiatric diagnoses

A number of studies have looked at parental psychiatric diagnoses other than depression and the association with childhood disturbance. Lee and Gotlib (1989) compared children of a group of depressed mothers to children of non-depressed psychiatric out-patients, including personality and anxiety disorders, and children of medical patients. The children of the depressed mothers appeared most impaired, but only slightly greater than the psychiatric out-patients; it was proposed that the degree of maternal psychopathology rather than the diagnosis was crucial in determining the child's outcome. Quinton and Rutter (1985) demonstrated that parental mental disorder was particularly damaging if in association with adverse psychosocial circumstances. Both in this study, and in Weissman et al's study (1984), personality disorders were linked to childhood conduct disorders, particularly where the child had been exposed to hostility. Hostility may, of course, go hand in hand with marital disorder, which was found in particular to be a mediating factor in childhood disorders.

Few studies have looked at children of anorexic mothers, although the higher incidence of relatives with eating and affective disorders is well known. Brinch et al (1988) followed up 151 patients with anorexia after 12 years; none of the 11 males had had children, and 50 of the women had had children. The outcome of these mothers was considered better than those who had remained childless, suggesting that those women able to have a relationship and a child had less psychopathology. Prematurity and prenatal morbidity were increased, compared to the normal population. Eight of the 75 children were less than 12 months of age, and assessment of the others was not adequate. However, 17% had failure to thrive in the first year of life and 9% had psychiatric disorder.

While these studies suggest maternal psychiatric illness and the associated psychosocial problems affect children, we still know very little about the crucial factors in the association: why some children are affected and not others, and what interventions might assist these children to develop normally. More studies are needed to help us understand this very complex area.

Case example

Jan, 24, was referred to a paediatrician by her general practitioner with her 5-month-old infant, who had failure to thrive. When first seen, although on the fiftieth percentile at birth, Crystal was now on the third. Investigations revealed no cause, and a psychiatric referral was made.

Jan had a history of prolonged sexual abuse and emotional neglect. As a child, she had a history of failure to thrive and subsequent untreated anorexia nervosa. Her relationship with her husband was strained and distant; they argued frequently over her lack of sexual interest.

Jan's first child had died of spina bifida at the age of 3 months. She immediately became pregnant again—that child, a boy, was aged 18 months and well. Crystal was also planned and had been well at birth, but Jan had feared throughout the pregnancy that the child would have spina bifida and still believed she might have a neurological deficit.

Jan, at first presentation, was a plump, pleasant woman whom it was difficult not to like. Crystal was a fragile-looking infant who smiled engagingly and rarely cried. Jan called her 'Fatso' and appeared unconcerned about her lack of weight: 'I was that thin at her age'.

Over many months of in-patient and out-patient therapy, a complex system evolved. When Jan was able to focus her own and medical staff's attention on Crystal, Jan remained well. Whenever her issues were focused on, she became severely depressed. A seesaw developed, where Jan would become depressed, and then Crystal would 'rescue' her by failing to put on weight. This issue was successfully addressed by nursing staff feeding the baby, resulting in marked weight gain. Jan also lost weight herself, and then no longer focused on this; Crystal became 'sick' instead. A variety of paediatric consultations and intervention followed.

Jan was able to present convincingly; she appeared to believe in these illnesses herself. Crystal she saw as being like herself; and there appeared to be a strong deep-seated compulsion to emotionally neglect Crystal as Jan herself had been neglected by her mother.

Individual and couple sessions were essential. Mother-infant sessions required a focus on Jan separating herself from Crystal, and being able to see Crystal as an individual, and her own issues quite separately. Long-term work is anticipated.

CHAPTER 8

Biological treatment

Aetiology

A biological basis for puerperal disorders has been proposed by many researchers.

Marked endocrine change occurs throughout pregnancy, and following delivery, during lactation and in the postpartum period. It has been an attractive proposition to link these changes with the mood disorders in the postpartum, but conclusive studies have remained elusive.

The hormonal changes that have been particularly focused on are the rapid decline in progesterone (Yalom et al 1968) and oestrogen (Weick et al 1991). Oestrogen has been shown to affect dopaminergic transmission in the central nervous system and the rapid decline in oestrogen after delivery may cause a hypersensitivity of hypothalamic dopamine receptors (Weick et al 1991). Henderson et al (1991) have shown some support for the use of oestradiol patches in severe postpartum depression. Klaiber et al (1979) suggested that the success of oestrogen treatment in their group of women with prolonged depression may have been related to effects on monoamine oxidase activity.

Progesterone has been used prophylactically for postpartum depression by Dalton (1983). Harris et al (1989b) suggested a link between low progesterone and depression in women who breastfeed, but a high level of progesterone in those bottle feeding. Gard et al (1986) found no association between mood in pregnancy or the puerperium with oestrogen or progesterone levels.

Links between premenstrual syndrome and postpartum depression have added weight to the theory of a hormonal basis. Pitt (1968), Yalom et al (1968), Tonge (1984) and Dennerstein et al (1989) found a history of premenstrual mood changes predictive of postpartum depression. O'Hara's (1987) conflicting findings may be a result of the method of assessment and the definition of premenstrual syndrome. Further evidence suggesting a hormonal aetiology comes from Dennerstein et al (1989), with findings linking continued total breastfeeding and depression. The difference in risk for those who totally breastfeed compared to those who supplement breastfeeding suggests the depression may be associated with the higher prolactin and/or lower oestrogen and progesterone found in those who totally breastfeed.

Lower androsterone and testosterone levels have also been found (Alder et al 1986). The observation in one study of a higher incidence of the 'blues' in the mothers of male infants led to the proposal that foetal testosterone withdrawal from the maternal circulation may be implicated (Tonge 1986), but this does not account for the 'blues' in mothers of female infants.

Cortisol has been noted to increase through pregnancy and labour and subsequently fall, most likely as a physiological response to the stress of childbirth (Steiner 1990). The finding that cortisol is elevated in response to dexamethasone suppression in people with depression is well known (Carroll 1972); however, it is difficult to evaluate postpartum as up to 80% dexamethasone suppression tests are positive (non-suppressed) up to 1 week postpartum (Steiner et al 1986). Handley et al (1980) found a slight association between postpartum depression and high cortisol at 38 weeks gestation but this was not replicated in a later study (Gard et al 1986).

Thyroid hormones have also been a focus. Harris et al (1992) found an association between depression and positive thyroid antibody status. They recommend that these women should be identified and monitored carefully.

Why these hormonal changes occur or affect some women but not others is unclear. It may be that there is a genetic predisposition: an association between puerperal psychiatric disorder and a past or family psychiatric history has been reported in a number of studies (Reich & Winokur 1970; Paykel et al 1980; Kendell 1985; Dennerstein et al 1989). This predisposition may also be what is triggered in recurrences of schizophrenia, bipolar disorder and some anxiety disorders that occur postpartum.

Biological intervention in postpartum disorders

In contrast to the many studies of the management of depression, no controlled study exists of the management of postpartum disorders (O'Hara & Zekoski 1988; Gitlin & Pasnau 1989). The tendency has been to categorise it under a general terminology (such as major depressive illness) and manage it accordingly (Steiner 1990).

While this approach is generally sound, it fails to consider some important issues:

The risk to the infant

The infant is exposed to medication given during pregnancy and while breast-feeding. This is discussed more fully at the end of this chapter and in the next.

Atypical presentation

Many women, often with quite severe depressive illnesses, may present initially quite well. They try hard to put up a front, to defend themselves against friends and families who expect them to be happy, or who offer well meant but ill-placed observations such as 'Of course you'll cope—I did', or 'You've only 1—I had 5 under the age of 6'. Depression in this period is the antithesis of what society and the woman expects; this appears to fuel the need to cover up such ill-timed feelings.

Common symptoms of major depression may not occur in depression postpartum. Sleep disturbance may be blamed on the infant, when often the woman lies awake quite independently of her child's feeding and waking patterns.

Lowered mood may be less prominent than lability (Oppenheim 1983), and appetite often disturbed but not necessarily lowered (Oppenheim 1983; Pauleikhoff 1987).

Postpartum depression then presents a problem to the clinician of under-recognition, because it may differ in presentation to depression at other times in the life cycle. The decision that medication is indicated may also not be straightforward. Reported symptom indicators for response to tricyclic antidepressants, which include weight loss, middle and late insomnia, psychomotor retardation, anhedonia and self-blame (Bielski & Friedel 1976; Tilley et al 1982), may not be evident. Severity of illness has been suggested as another indicator of potential therapeutic response to tricyclic antidepressants (Bielski & Friedel 1976). However, observer-rated scales such as the Hamilton Depression Rating Scales that are non-specific and non-standardised in the postpartum period are usually suggested as indicators of severity (Hamilton 1967). The only specific tool for this period, the Edinburgh Postnatal Depression Scale, is for screening and not for severity assessment (Cox et al 1987).

Given this atypical presentation, depression can go unrecognised and the severity be under-diagnosed.

Keller et al (1982) comment that many depressed patients, for whom antidepressants are indicated, do not receive them or, when they do, do not receive adequate doses. This is even more likely in postpartum depression.

If the woman is pregnant or breastfeeding this may further influence the treating doctor not to commence or increase treatment. Electroconvulsive therapy (ECT) may not be considered. Despite its negative image, ECT still has a role in the management of postpartum psychosis and severe postpartum depression. It can give a dramatic response. It needs to be considered in situations where the woman is suicidal, is deteriorating and/or has not responded to medication.

It is crucial not to miss the mild or moderate disorders, and also not to under-treat the mild, moderate or severe disorders. Broader issues, other than biological treatments, need to be addressed in all cases.

Risks to the infant need to be considered but not to treat the disorder aggressively is a *far greater risk* to the woman, her partner, the viability of the relationship and the long-term development of her child.

Case example

Jane, a 24-year-old secretary, was seen by her general practitioner on an increasing number of occasions over the first 3 months postpartum. She was diagnosed as having maternal exhaustion and admitted reluctantly for a week to a mother-baby hospital. She was observed to be withdrawn, tearful and relieved to hand over care of her child, a son who had been unplanned but wanted. Her husband, a nursing orderly, was supportive but worked long hours in two jobs for financial reasons. There were no family supports and she lived in an isolated area.

Jane was begun on dothiepin, up to 150 mg/d, but failed to improve. She attended her general practitioner irregularly, and stopped taking the medication, feeling the situation was hopeless. Her husband encouraged her to attend a mental health clinic, but this meant travelling a long distance on public transport, and due to expenditure cuts her appointments were brief and with different doctors. After brief trials of inadequate doses of antidepressants over inadequate time periods, she again stopped taking medication. Jane's depression continued, and she also experienced chronic pelvic pain and dysmenorrhea. At 27 she opted for an elective hysterectomy. Six months later she had a severe major depressive illness, which was untreated. She rarely left the house; her son spent most days sitting directly in front of the television. On a range of cognitive scales his performance was markedly retarded.

Cases such as this are fortunately not common, but they do occur. They may occur more often than realised; this woman came to attention only because of her agreement at 3 months postpartum to be part of a research study. Her isolation, her lack of family support and the hopelessness that was part of her illness, were aggravating factors. Aggressive treatment, follow-up of appointments not kept, and a domiciliary team could have helped her, and her child's, outcome, to be far more positive.

Choice of drug

The choice of medication will depend initially on diagnosis.

Psychotic illness in the postpartum period frequently has affective symptoms and a combination of major tranquillisers and antidepressants may be required. The presentation of mania is usually followed by depression; in these cases antidepressants may not be required initially. For women with a history of psychotic illness, the medication to which response has been previously noted is likely to be the drug of first choice.

In both psychotic and depressive illnesses, anxiety and agitation may be a major feature. This can be unsettling for the infant, and interferes with the developing relationship. Sedation in these situations is often preferable. Major tranquillisers such as thioridazine and chlorpromazine can work quickly and effectively. For depression with a high level of anxiety, a sedative tricyclic such as amitriptyline is appropriate and minimises the need for concurrent use of minor tranquillisers.

When beginning any sedative for an out-patient it is important to do so slowly, and to have a family member available to feed and care for the infant if the mother is unable to do so. In a hospital, trained nursing staff need to be available for this role.

For many women, however, being available and alert for the night feeds is essential and excessive sedation is inappropriate. Women who are breastfeeding may be particularly reluctant to persevere with excessive sedation if it interferes with this special role.

Current Australian practice (Buist 1994) favours the use of dothiepin as the first-line treatment. Our experience is that it is well tolerated and that the mild sedation helps the anxiety and assists with sleep without interfering with night feeds.

Other newer antidepressants may also be of benefit. Lack of energy is a frequent component of postpartum depression and the lack of sedation and the energising qualities of these newer drugs are likely to benefit these women. Moclobemide, thought to be useful for depression with concurrent anxiety, may be particularly beneficial. A study is under way evaluating its effectiveness (Dennerstein et al). With the SSRIs (selective serotonin reuptake inhibitors) our experience is that the agitation is initially heightened by fluoxetine and this is intolerable for many; some women do well on this, however. The newer drugs, sertraline and paroxetine, look more promising.

Hormones

Research has sought a hormonal basis for postpartum disorders (and continues to do so), but studies have failed to demonstrate a conclusive link. Adequate, controlled trials in the use of oestrogen or progesterone have yet to be published. There are some promising early studies, but these are not adequate to justify the use of hormonal treatments, at least as a first-line treatment; however, for women who have failed to respond to traditional antidepressant treatments, particularly where there is no significant psychosocial component to their disorder, augmentation with oestradiol patches is worth considering. Reports from trials using oestradiol patches for prevention and treatment have been disappointing. Until adequate trials have been reported, low doses are recommended: the effects of oestrogen, particularly on the lactating breast, are largely unknown, and the possible cancer risk reported in some menopausal studies raises cause for concern. Studies using oestradiol have required heparinisation, and thus it is unsuitable for standard clinical practice.

In these women, testing of thyroid status is also appropriate; results of the use of thyroxine in depressed women with thyroid antibodies and borderline thyroid function have yet to be published (Harris et al 1992).

Pregnancy and the use of medication

Most drug companies do not advocate taking psychotropic medication in pregnancy, but women with psychiatric disorders on medication may become pregnant, and psychiatric disorders occur antenatally. There is concern regarding teratogenicity and complications at term, but few studies have addressed this. Most reports are case reports and anecdotal evidence. A review of current knowledge follows.

Mood stabilisers

Lithium needs to be avoided in the first trimester, and all women treated with this drug should be using adequate contraception and warned of the risks (Mortola 1989; Sitland-Marken et al 1989). In the first several years of the International Register of Lithium, of the 225 babies reported, 7 babies were stillborn and 25 had major congenital malformations (Schou & Weinstein 1980). Of the 25 with major malformations, 18 involved the heart and great vessels, including 6 with Ebstein's anomaly. Most of these cases were born to mothers who received lithium in the first trimester. As well, toxicity has been noted in some newborns of mothers who had taken lithium at term (Ananth 1975). Jacobson et al (1992) have suggested that the risk may not be as high as previously thought, but the suspicion is that lithium should be avoided where possible. Where an unplanned pregnancy occurs, the potential risks need to be explained: the decision to continue or not with pregnancy is a difficult one and requires support from the prescribing doctor. A summary of the use of lithium during pregnancy and lactation has been presented by Linden and Rich (1983), and strategies for the management of acute mania have been presented by Sitland-Marken et al (1989).

Lithium in the second and third trimester should be used with caution, and its levels monitored closely, particularly at term, when there are rapid alterations in fluid balance and changes in glomerular filtration rate. Higher doses required in pregnancy can quickly lead to toxicity postpartum, so doses should be divided and tapered towards term.

Carbamazepine, also used as a mood stabiliser, should also be avoided in the first trimester, as there is evidence of major abnormality and spina bifida (Jones et al 1991; Rosa 1991). Verapamil, found to be of use in some patients who have not responded to the mood stabilisers, has been found to decrease uterine blood flow and reduce foetal arterial oxygen centrally so it should also be avoided throughout pregnancy.

Antidepressants

A few larger studies looking at antidepressants in pregnancy exist. Large-scale reviews of birth defects and pregnancies have found no link with foetal deformities (Crombie et al 1975; Kuenssberg & Knox 1972; Idanpaan-Heikkla & Saxen 1973).

Pastusak et al (1993) looked at 128 pregnant women exposed to a mean dose of 25.8 mg of fluoxetine in the first trimester and compared them to women using tricyclics. They concluded that neither fluoxetine nor tricyclics showed evidence of teratogenicity, but that both were associated with higher rates of miscarriage (13.5% fluoxetine and 12.2% tricyclic compared to 6.8% controls).

An evaluation by Goldstein and Williams (1992) of 239 pregnant women exposed to fluoxetine concluded that there was no evidence of teratogenicity nor increased risk of miscarriage, but reported an increase in hyper-bilirubinaemia and jitteriness in the neonate.

Case reports of paroxetine in pregnancy give no evidence of teratogenicity.

Monoamines are generally avoided because of risks of concomitant toxaemia and anaesthetic complications of an emergency delivery (Mortola 1989). This cannot be said of moclobemide, about which little is known.

Anxiolytics

Conflicting findings have been reported regarding benzodiazepines in pregnancy. A higher incidence of oral clefts was reported by Saffra and Oakley (1975) but not by Shiono and Mills (1984); in both cases numbers were very small. Eight children exposed to high doses of diazepam in utero were reported to have dysmorphic features, growth retardation and central nervous system abnormalities (Laegreid et al 1975). Two studies found a higher risk of perinatal death (Laegreid et al 1975; Pasker-de Jong et al 1992). Little data is available specifically on clonazepam (Czeizel et al 1992). Little data is also available about anxiolytics other than benzodiazepines. Propranolol has been thought to cause intra-uterine growth retardation (Eliahov et al 1978). Dose-related growth retardation, oral clefts and skeletal abnormalities have been noted with barbiturates (Heinonen et al 1977). Withdrawal symptoms, hypotonia and poor sucking have been noted in newborns exposed to diazepam or barbiturates in pregnancy, and this may last for some weeks (Robinson et al 1986).

Major tranquillisers

Some studies (Rumeau-Roquette et al 1977; Edlund & Craig 1984) have suggested possible teratogenic effects of phenothiazines, but most do not reveal significant foetal abnormalities in the infants of women taking phenothiazines or butyrophenones (Slone et al 1977; Milkovich & Van den Berg 1976; Goldberg & Di Mascio 1978; Ananth 1975). However, effects of factors such as dose, other medications, smoking and maternal age need to be considered and the findings of these studies are not conclusive. An extrapyramidal syndrome has been reported in infants exposed to chlorpromazine near term (Hill et al 1966; Ayd 1968; O'Connor et al 1981).

Case example

Theresa, 32, presented to an antenatal clinic for her first appointment at 36 weeks gestation. It was her sixth pregnancy and she had 4 children in foster care, from 3 different partners. The father of this child was unknown. Her first psychiatric contact had been at 8 years old, and she had had many subsequent admissions, her most recent 4 years earlier, at which time her diagnosis was borderline intellectual impairment and chronic schizophrenia. At this time she had been treated with fluoxetine 60 mg/d, pericyazine 30 mg/d and oxazepam 90 mg/d. Her medication had stayed the same, despite regular attendances at the local mental health clinic.

At 36 weeks gestation, Theresa presented with psychomotor retardation and vegetative symptoms of depression, largely consistent with excessive sedation. She was admitted to hospital and the medication withdrawn. There was initial improvement, which was more marked following delivery. The infant, a full-term 3690 g (8lb 2oz) girl, had a low apgar score, was noted to be floppy and to suck poorly. There were soft neurological signs present. She required nasogastric feeding for the first 2 months of life. Thorough investigation revealed no cause for this; exposure to high doses of medication throughout pregnancy, and the fluoxetine which would still have been present at birth due to its long half-life, was thought most likely responsible. Clearly, Theresa's medication should have been reviewed by the mental health clinic at her first disclosure of pregnancy, not in her final weeks.

Theresa's depressive and psychotic symptoms re-emerged postpartum; they responded well to amitriptyline 225 mg/d and thioridazine 300 mg/d. These were chosen in view of her high levels of anxiety. She remained well on this in hospital, but she returned to minor tranquillisers abuse after discharge.

Conclusions

In view of the lack of data, psychotropic use in pregnancy needs to be considered cautiously. Some medications, as detailed previously, should be avoided. Women who have a history of psychiatric disorder and who are already on medication need a critical review of their management. Where possible, medication should be avoided in the first trimester. Doses should be kept to the minimum and tapered towards term. Where higher doses are required, probably due to the altered metabolism and excretion during pregnancy, close monitoring of the foetus is essential.

CHAPTER 9

Breastfeeding

Breastfeeding attitudes

Postpartum depression and psychosis usually have an onset within the first 6 weeks postpartum (Kumar & Robson 1984). During this time and subsequently, many women are breastfeeding their babies. Breastfeeding has the advantages for the mother of simplicity and portability, with no expense, and the provision of some contraceptive protection (Cunningham 1981; Ferry & Smith 1983). For the baby the milk composition is tailored to organ development with nutritional and immunological superiority. It is associated with less obesity and decreased morbidity of the infant (Wilson et al 1980; Kocturk & Zetterstrom 1988; Williamen 1989).

Breastfeeding also carries no risk of the type of infections with which bottle feeding and the water sterilisation of bottles have been associated, although maternal exposure to drugs and contaminates may be a contraindication to breastfeeding (Ford & Labhok 1990). Breastfeeding also contributes to the bond between mother and child (Williamen 1989).

These benefits are particularly important to women and their children in developing countries (Kocturk & Zetterstrom 1988).

There has been a strong promotion of breastfeeding in recent years, particularly by community groups such as the Nursing Mothers' Association of Australia (Bundrock 1989). The sharp decline in breastfeeding in the 1930s through to the 1960s, attributed to the introduction of infant formulas, resulted in World Health Organisation recommendations which have precipitated a dramatic subsequent increase in breastfeeding in the Western world (Kocturk & Zetterstrom 1988).

Eighty-five per cent of Australian mothers begin breastfeeding (Bundrock 1989), although some stop within the first month; factors such as sore nipples, maternal fatigue, inadequate supply and 'violated expectations' are cited as reasons (Kearney et al 1990; Crepman et al 1985).

In other industrialised countries the numbers of breastfeeding women are not as great. In the US, 60% of mothers begin breastfeeding (Ford & Labhok 1990), and in New Zealand 70% of mothers begin breastfeeding (Msuya et al 1990).

In an international study, 74% of Australian women, 32% of Dutch women and 44% of Italian women were breastfeeding 4 months after delivery (Dennerstein et al 1989). The Australian figure was higher than that of a subsequent review which probably reflects sample selection. In Victoria, a Health Department review (1990) found 57% of women were breastfeeding at 3 months and 42% at 6 months, an increase by a factor of 5 since 1971.

Women who continue to breastfeed are in general better educated, tend to be older, more affluent, have greater perceived support and longer intended duration of feeding (Kocturk & Zetterstrom 1988; Williamen 1989; John & Mattarel 1989; Ford & Labhok 1990; Kearney et al 1990). The encouragement to breastfeed arguably has the most impact on women whose education encourages reading, attending classes, and consulting opinions from the health profession; these have a considerable influence, although not always a helpful one (Lowe 1990).

Association of breastfeeding with depression

Breastfeeding and depression are important issues to be considered together.

Firstly, breastfeeding, by its effect on the woman's hormonal status, may be associated aetiologically. Continued total breastfeeding has been linked with lowered mood and libido at up to 4 months postpartum (Alder et al 1986; Alder & Bancroft 1988; Dennerstein et al 1989), although this may disappear by 6 months (Alder & Bancroft 1988).

There are a number of possible explanations for this relationship. The finding may be related to lower gonadal hormones or the higher prolactin found in women who breastfeed (Alder et al 1986; Harris et al 1989b). Alder and Cox (1983) found that among a group of 62 breastfeeding women, those with normal levels of endogenous hormones were the least likely to have depressive symptoms. Alder and Bancroft (1988) noted that breastfeeding had more effect on sexuality than mood, and proposed that the practical consequences of breastfeeding may have been an important factor, and that the apparent negative effects of breastfeeding were likely to be multifactorial. The physical tie to the infant may be a factor in some women.

In Harris et al's study (1989b), lower prolactin levels were noted in depressed breastfeeding women compared to those breastfeeding who were not depressed. Numbers in this study were small, however, and statistical significance was only on the Edinburgh Postnatal Depression Scale (Cox et al 1987).

Studies on postpartum blues looking at prolactin levels have given conflicting results. Steiner et al (1986) found women with the blues were more likely to have lower prolactin levels, but this has not been replicated by others (Mendlewicz et al 1980; Judd et al 1982).

Other explanations for the association of total breastfeeding and low mood include lower androstenedione (Alder et al 1986), which is higher in those who partially breastfeed and who appear at less risk of depression. This appears to be only one of many factors that might be contributing to the postpartum depression.

Secondly, the impact of maternal depression on the woman needs consideration in the on-going management decision whether to breastfeed. Milk supply may be inadequate secondary to anxiety and stress (Tamminen 1988). Depressed women are more likely to have difficulties tolerating the problems that may occur, and are less likely to have the positive attitude, low anxiety and increased confidence associated with those women who continue to breastfeed (Kearney et al 1990). A decision to stop breast-feeding may be regretted later, and may be in conflict with the woman and her family's idealised attitudes and education that says 'breast is best'. Cessation of breastfeeding may jeopardise the bonding, and add to the sense of failure.

Those who do wish to stop may find difficulties in asserting themselves against well-meaning family and professionals. For some women, the demands and dependence of the breastfed baby is an added psychosocial stress, precluding family assistance and use of daycare or crèche facilities. The permission to stop may be a relief.

Finally, the depressed woman who requires medication and who is breastfeeding faces not only the dilemmas mentioned, but also the risk to her baby from medication excreted in breast milk.

Many women express concern about the effects of drugs on their infant. Community attitudes have moved away from unquestioned acceptance of the doctor's opinion and such social pressures influence individual decisions. Yet, while psychotropic medication has been in use for, in some cases, over 30 years, there is a great paucity of information available on the effects of these medications in pregnancy and on breastfed infants. On the other hand, it should be remembered that an increasing number of studies are linking breastfeeding to improved cognitive development.

Breastfeeding and the use of medication

Case reports on the use of psychotropic medication while breastfeeding have been reviewed in an earlier article (Buist et al 1990). These revealed a lack of controlled studies with most of the literature being merely individual case reports. Only the most basic conclusions can be drawn from animal studies. There are ethical and moral difficulties in studying drug effects in the nursing mother, and in setting up experimental and control groups. Chemical studies on the milk and plasma are complicated.

Maternal pharmacokinetics and the transport of the drug into the milk are affected by drug solubility and frequency of any administration, as well as any absorption, blood flow and breast metabolism. The young infant is a rapidly changing entity whose metabolism and excretion of drugs alters quickly (Knowles 1965; O'Brien 1974; Wilson et al 1980). Responses cannot be predicted according to an adult model.

Many studies have not taken these factors into account, and drug levels have frequently been measured before a steady state has been achieved. In general, these medications do pass into breast milk, although the level to which the infant is exposed may be low. Both short and long-term further studies need to be conducted before any firm conclusions can be drawn.

Mood stabilisers

Lithium is excreted in human breast milk (Tunnessen & Hertz 1972; Schou & Amdisen 1973; Sykes et al 1976). In one case the mother had been treated with lithium throughout the pregnancy (Tunnessen & Hertz 1972). At birth the baby was hypotonic and cyanosed. The baby subsequently improved, but deteriorated again when breastfeeding was begun. Serum lithium levels were 1.5 mmol/L in the mother and 0.6 mmol/L in the infant at 5 days of age, while breast milk levels were the same as the infant's serum levels.

In contrast, maternal and infant serum levels were reported as similar in another case where the mother was maintained on 400 mg/d of lithium (Sykes et al 1976). Concentrations of lithium in the infant continued to fall over 2 weeks despite increasing maternal serum and breast-milk concentrations as well as increasing the dose. The milk/plasma ratio of lithium decreased from 0.77 to 0.25 from day 28 to day 42, suggesting that factors other than serum concentration determine the amount of lithium in breast milk.

Schou and Amdisen (1973) reported 8 cases of children breastfed by women receiving lithium treatment. The milk/plasma ratio varied from 0.24 to 0.67; that is similar to that reported by Sykes and co-workers. Concentrations in the mother's serum were 1.5 to 5.6 times those in the child's serum. No firm conclusions were drawn regarding the safety of continuing to breastfeed during lithium therapy. On the one hand it was noted that exposure to low levels in breast milk would be unlikely to do any harm, yet any unnecessary exposure to drugs is undesirable. In later statements Schou thought it advisable that women should bottle feed, not breastfeed their children (Schou & Vestergaard 1983). This recommendation was prompted by the sensitivity of the kidneys to lithium, in particular morphological changes with chronic administration. Coupled with the propensity for goitre or myxoedema and a diabetes-insipidus-like syndrome caused by long-term lithium exposure, this recommendation would appear clinically prudent.

Antidepressants

Isolated cases of possible toxic effects in breastfed infants whose mothers have been on doxepin (Matheson et al 1985) have been reported.

A more detailed study of 20 women taking dothiepin (Buist et al 1993) showed the drug did pass into breast milk, with considerable individual variation, as has been observed in plasma. Similar levels were found in breast milk to that in the plasma. No problems were observed in the infant. A recent follow-up study (Buist and Janson, in press) found no effects at 3 to 5 years on the cognitive performance of these children, compared to infants of depressed mothers who had not been exposed to medication. It is likely that these findings would be true of other tricyclics also; but numbers were small and the finding should be regarded with caution. There are no other long-term studies yet reported.

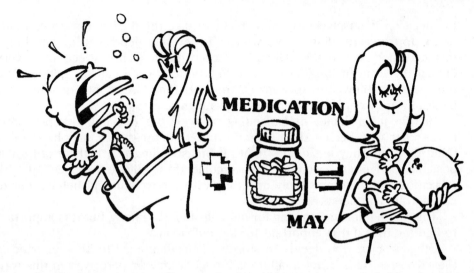

In a small study of 15, no cognitive effects were found in children 3 to 5 years who had been breastfed while the mother was on dothiepin

Little work has been done on the newer antidepressants. Fluoxetine needs to be considered warily because of its long half-life. Case reports have suggested moclobemide is excreted in very small amounts only; but these were after single doses and steady state had not been achieved.

Anxiolytics

Diazepam has been found to be excreted into breast milk, with the risk of lethargy in the infant (Erkkola & Kanto 1972). Small doses may not be a problem but the infant should be observed closely for sedation and secondary feeding difficulties and failure to thrive. Matheson et al (1990) looked at midazolam and nitrazepam used as nocturnal sedation and found no detectable levels of the former; milk concentrations of nitrazepam increased with regular use. They concluded that the use of these minor tranquillisers as night sedation was probably safe.

Major tranquillisers

Like other medications, major tranquillisers are excreted into breast milk, usually in small concentrations. Isolated case reports of sedation and toxicity in infants have been reported (Wilson et al 1980); low doses have been thought to be safe (Mortola 1989).

Breastfeeding—management issues

Breastfeeding has different psychological meaning for each individual. If medication is required, it is essential that the woman and her family are given a thorough explanation of any potential risks, and ample time to make the decision themselves—to take or not to take the medication, to continue or to stop breastfeeding. If the woman is severely depressed or psychotic, this may not be possible. Often in these situations breastfeeding is very difficult because of the illness itself. Psychotic women can be agitated and the infant not allowed to suck for an adequate time. Breast milk quantity may be significantly depleted where anxiety is high.

On the other hand, breastfeeding may be the one link the psychotic mother has with her child; in women who are depressed, it may be the one thing they feel they are doing 'right'. If breastfeeding is a high priority it is possible, and often essential, to overcome these difficulties, helping with relaxation and building supply or sitting with the woman and helping her to concentrate and persevere.

This can be time-consuming for nursing staff and family, but it is important to find the time if it is important to that individual.

Other women who decide to stop breastfeeding need to be supported in their decision. This is not a failure, although it may be perceived in this way. Challenging this perception can be included in cognitive therapy, helping the woman herself to challenge and respond to negative beliefs such as this.

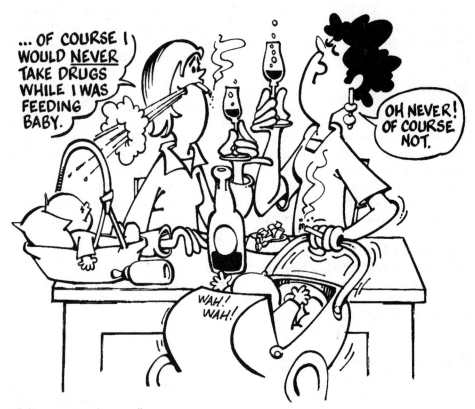

All drugs pass into breast milk

For those women who continue breastfeeding and taking medication, the infant needs to be observed closely, particularly in the early stages, but also for any evidence of accumulation. Where there is concern, measurement of levels in the breast milk or the infant can be generally available in most major cities. Further studies are looking at a number of medications and potential long-term effects on the development of the child.

Case example

Margerita, a 28-year-old pathology technician, was admitted with postpartum depression with her infant at 2 weeks postpartum. The pregnancy was planned and went normally. Birth was uncomplicated. Her husband, Ross, a teacher, was supportive of his wife but reluctant for her to be admitted, and adamant that she continue breastfeeding. They both had strong views on childbirth being natural, and breast milk being best for the child. Over the subsequent week her depression escalated. She became withdrawn, hostile and suspicious, keeping to her room and rarely speaking spontaneously. On questioning, she indicated that she felt the staff wished to harm her. She also admitted to suicidal ideas and had planned to jump from the top of the hospital. On this occasion she was found heading towards the stairs.

Margerita was considered a serious suicidal risk. Because the ward had no secure facilities, moving her to a psychiatric hospital was discussed with her husband. He refused this, and ECT. We decided to give her a week trial of remaining on the ward, being 'specialled' during the day and having her husband stay with her overnight in our high-observation room. If she was still at risk at the end of the week, we felt there was no option but to certify her. We gave her this time to allow the antidepressants to work, and because the perceived stigma of certification, psychiatric hospitalisation and possible separation from her child would have been hugely traumatic to this family.

During this week, Margerita required intensive input of nursing and medical time. Although her husband (and she later) were concerned about the risks to their infant of the dothiepin, they felt the benefits of breastfeeding were greater. Breast milk levels were taken and moderately high levels noted. Blood samples were taken from the infant, in which the dothiepin was barely detectable. Over this time, Margerita was highly anxious, and worried that her infant was not getting adequate milk. She became delusional about this, denying that the child was gaining weight on test weighs and refusing to believe that her engorged leaking breasts had milk. She was reassured, and nursing staff reinforced the finding of weight gain. She breastfed for longer and more often than required, but during this time was affectionate, concerned and clearly loving towards her infant.

Dothiepin had been begun and was quickly increased to 225 mg. After 10 days on this dose, significant improvement was observed.

After a further week, Margerita was essentially her normal self, and her warm relationship with her infant prospered. She continued to breastfeed until the child was 1 year old, stopping when she wished to get pregnant again. Because of her rapid response and her eagerness to minimise the risk to her infant, she was maintained on dothiepin for only 3 months. She did not relapse and the child at 4 years has developed normally.

CHAPTER 10

In-patient and community management

Introduction

Psychiatric disorders in most instances can be managed on an out-patient basis with community supports. This is true, too, of postpartum psychiatric disorders—but where the sufferer is the primary caregiver for a dependent infant, the safety and welfare of the infant and the stress of being the caregiver need to be considered. Often the need for family and community supports is greater than their availability.

Counter-balancing these concerns is the prospect of hospitalisation breaking up the family, with possibly separation from the infant, and the associated perceived stigma of being admitted. Women are often already feeling a failure; for some, hospital can be an alien place that reinforces their guilt and despair.

When general practitioners, maternal-child health nurses and other professionals are confronted with this dilemma the decision is a difficult one. Wherever possible, the decision to be admitted or not should be the woman's, in conjunction with her partner, if present. Being made aware of what the local options are will help the family; visiting or talking to the referral agency may alleviate some anxiety.

When to refer

A patient should be referred:
1. if there is a risk of suicide;
2. if the infant, or older children, are at risk, either directly or through neglect;
3. if there is a psychotic illness;
4. if distress is excessive or prolonged, particularly where family and/or community supports are inadequate;

5. if symptoms have failed to respond to adequate out-patient treatment;
6. if assessment of parenting skills and safety issues is required.

Suicide risk

Women whose psychiatric disorders have been previously stable, or who are experiencing a psychiatric illness for the first time, can be overwhelmed by their feelings and the full-time dependency of their infant. Suicide is not common, but the wish to 'not wake up' is, and the suicide risk needs to be carefully evaluated and re-evaluated, particularly in women with severe depression and psychotic illnesses. Mood in bipolar illnesses can quickly swing; manic and depressive features are often apparent in postpartum psychosis. Whenever there is any concern, an assessment by a psychiatrist is essential.

Case example

Gwen, 33, was kept in hospital for 2 weeks after the birth of her first child, because of concerns that her mood was not stable. She had a history of bipolar disorder and had stopped taking lithium before becoming pregnant. She had not resumed lithium because of her desire to breastfeed. Her mood had been labile but there was no evidence of psychosis. Although anxious about caring for her child, she coped well. One morning she was noted to be withdrawn; at a later ward round she was unable to be found. Her baby was in the nursery. Some days later her body was identified on the river's edge. The coroner's verdict was death by drowning, most likely suicide.

This tragedy could probably not have been avoided, in view of the rapid mood swing, but it heightens the awareness of suicide potential in sufferers of bipolar disorder (and the awareness of how destabilising childbirth can be). There is a strong case for reinstating lithium where it has been previously effective, immediately post delivery, and foregoing breastfeeding.

Child at risk

The safety of dependent children is paramount. They cannot speak for themselves, and it is up to the treating health professionals to consider their safety. Psychiatric disorder does not, of course, make the sufferer dangerous; however, issues of safety may be twofold in postpartum disorders:
1. if the child is incorporated into a delusional system in a psychotic illness or severe depression; or
2. the woman is so severely affected that her judgment and concentration are impaired and the child or children are neglected or put at risk.

The longer-term issues are discussed in Chapter 7.

Women with postpartum depression frequently report that they have obsessional thoughts about harming their child. Some have intrusive images of knives, dropping the child or slipping while holding the child in the bath. They are distressed and guilt-ridden by such thoughts, and although they may fear doing such a thing, the fear is usually of the thought rather than of the reality. If they report such thoughts, it is important not to overreact and reinforce the guilt. Assessment by a psychiatrist is advisable. Not all women with these thoughts need to be admitted, but it is essential to establish how safe the woman herself feels. Therapy can help deal with these fears, often in conjunction with medication.

Case example – 1

Peggy, 27, was a single mother, self-referred to a mother-baby unit, feeling unable to cope with her 2-week-old daughter. She had a history of multiple admissions over the previous 10 years, where a history of childhood sexual abuse had been noted and a diagnosis of borderline personality disorder made. In the unit, she was demanding of staff time, argumentative and reluctant to accept responsibility for child care. A week after admission she became withdrawn, and suspicious of staff, claiming they were spying on her and trying to poison her. Later in the day she said she wished her baby was dead, and informed staff of a number of ways in which she planned to kill the child.

As the unit did not have secure facilities, and because it was felt that both Peggy and her infant were at risk, Peggy was sent as an involuntary patient to a psychiatric hospital. Protective services were informed and foster care arranged. Peggy's condition quickly settled; she was later reunited with her infant in a supervised environment. Subsequent custody depended on initial supervision.

Case example – 2

Jacqueline, 25, a married nurse, presented with a moderate depressive illness and marked anxiety. The anxiety was largely centred around her infant's health and her fear that she was an inadequate mother. She began having thoughts of stabbing her infant whenever dealing with the kitchen knives. These were recognised as her own thoughts, and ones which were unwelcome and caused great distress. She was adamant she would never harm her infant intentionally and was at a loss to understand these thoughts.

Jacqueline's depressive symptoms responded well to out-patient treatment of dothiepin 225 mg/d, but her thoughts continued, although in a diminished way. In therapy she realised that she resented being at home while her husband worked and, although she loved her infant, she had difficulties reconciling the role of mother with that of worker. With therapy and cognitive behavioural techniques the problem of the thoughts was fully resolved.

Psychotic illnesses

Even if there are no apparent suicide or infanticide risks, and there is a family member present to care for the child, most women with acute psychotic illnesses should be assessed and stabilised in hospital. Some illnesses will settle quickly, but others may be prolonged, unpredictable and unstable. In some areas, psychiatric crisis teams in conjunction with a supportive family may be able to keep these women at home, but as yet there is an inadequate number of intensive teams specialising in this area and this option is not readily available.

Case example

Jo, a 28-year-old teacher, was admitted at 2 weeks postpartum after increasing agitation and sleep disturbance, where she had woken neighbours and friends in the early hours of the morning. She admitted to auditory hallucinations of God speaking to her, and appeared confused and insightless. There was no history of previous psychiatric disorder, but a grandmother had had bipolar affective disorder. Her behaviour was too disruptive for her to remain at home and, although agreeable to admission, she was reluctant to accept medication and was erratic and at times behaved inappropriately with her child. She required hospitalisation for 6 months and was treated with a variety of antidepressants, major tranquillisers and ECT. She remained on medication until her child was 2, when she had returned to her normal self and to teaching.

Severity and inadequate supports

Psychiatric illness is distressing for the sufferer and her family at any time. So too, can be a young infant, who is dependent, unsettled and unpredictable. The combination of the two, over the weeks or months it may take the disorder to respond to treatment, can cause great anxiety. There may be frequent contact with a variety of agencies. Reassurance and support may be adequate—but not always. In particular, women without partners, or with partners who work interstate or for long hours, or who live in isolated areas, or with little extended family, may reach breaking point. Admission is preferable before this occurs.

Case example

Noelene, 17, was admitted, after many crisis calls, with her 4-month-old infant. Her 17-year-old boyfriend Tim spent significant time in the unit with her. Noelene had been a street kid since running away from her family home, where she had been raped by her stepfather. There was no contact with her family, and Tim's family had disowned them both when she had become pregnant. At the time of admission the child was well cared for, but Noelene expressed fears about her and Tim's ability to continue in their relationship and as parents. The admission allowed this couple 'time-out' in a supportive environment, giving them time and guidance to look at options and re-evaluate strengths in their relationship. At discharge Noelene had a part-time job and had organised child care, which would continue the following year when she planned to study, and they had been linked in with other young, local parents.

Treatment failure

There may be a variety of reasons why an illness fails to respond to treatment, including incorrect diagnosis, inadequate doses or duration of medication, noncompliance, concomitant use of non-prescription drugs or psychosocial stresses of which the clinician is unaware. Admission can clarify these issues.

Case example

Danielle, a 25-year-old mother of 2, failed to respond to adequate treatment trials of 2 antidepressants. She maintained that she had no current stresses but her blanket, 'too-bright' denial aroused suspicion and she was admitted. For the first week she was polite, distant and moderately depressed. On the first weekend her de facto arrived intoxicated to collect her and became violent. Danielle admitted that his alcohol problem had escalated since the birth of their last child. Major issues emerged in the partnership, and also in her relationship with her mother. Once she was able to admit these problems, work initially as an in-patient and then longer term as an out-patient allowed a slow but steady improvement.

Parenting assessment

The capacity to be a parent is not inherent. For some women, with a history of intellectual impairment or psychiatric disorder, concerns may exist about their ability to care for an infant. These concerns may be generated by family, hospital maternity staff or by other health professionals. Protective services may have become involved before the child's birth, or have been contacted subsequently. In this situation, an in-patient admission may be the quickest and safest option in order to assess the situation. An admission can also provide education in child care; referral following birth can help disadvantaged women have a smoother transition to motherhood.

Case example

May, a 24-year-old single woman with a 7-year history of schizophrenia, had had protective services involved by her general practitioner during the pregnancy. May's illness responded well to major tranquillisers, but she was noncompliant in taking medication and itinerant with no family supports. Postpartum, she and her infant were assessed in a mother-baby unit. It had been thought unlikely that she would be able to care for a child. On admission, her acute psychotic symptoms had settled, but she had difficulty motivating herself to get out of bed and had only limited insight into the dependency of her infant. Nevertheless, she was warm to, and caring of, her infant. In view of her difficulties when in the unit, and past history of noncompliance, on-going concern was noted, but a strong recommendation to keep mother and infant together was made. A longer-term placement was arranged for her and her child in a group home where supervision was available.

Where to refer

Since Main (1985) first proposed that women and their infants be admitted together in 1948, 'mother-baby' units have been established throughout the United Kingdom, and more recently in Australia (Buist et al 1990; Fowler & Brandon 1965; Lindsay 1975; Kissane & Ball 1988). It has been thought that they would prevent disruption to the mother–infant relationship, and help promote the woman's confidence as a mother, allowing her to deal with the stress of being a caregiver in a supportive environment. Grouping women together can also provide a supportive environment and intensive specialised input.

Mother-baby units may exist:
1. in psychiatric hospitals;
2. in psychiatric wards of general hospitals;
3. in psychiatric wards of private hospitals; and
4. in obstetric hospitals.

Some psychiatric wards will allow a baby to accompany a mother, but have no mother-baby unit as such. This allows the mother to remain with the infant but hasn't the other advantages. Staff in psychiatric wards are rarely experienced in dealing with an infant in this setting and such admissions may produce considerable anxiety. Although the presence of an infant is usually greeted positively by other patients (Glaser 1962), the safety of the infant

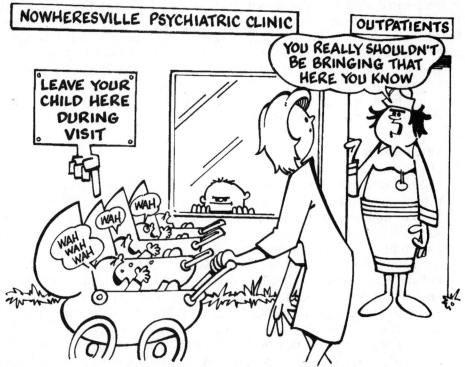

Mother-baby units ... prevent disruption to the mother–infant relationship

needs to be considered. One report was of an infant fatality caused by another non-postpartum patient, not by the mother (Bardon et al 1968).

After-care hospitals may also accept women with milder psychiatric disorders.

In some localities admission with a baby may not be possible. Where infanticide is a risk, it is advisable not to admit mother and infant together, at least in the early phases.

Availability will largely dictate where a referral is made. Although units have been in psychiatric hospitals in the past, the current trend towards mainstreaming means that obstetric and general hospital admissions will become more likely in the future.

The Mercy Hospital for Women Mother-Baby Unit optimises this trend, and was opened largely in response to the demands of patients themselves to be kept with their infants, and in a setting where a perceived stigma is minimal. Having a unit within an obstetric setting has many advantages. Continuity of care through pregnancy and the postpartum is streamlined, with access to obstetric, paediatric and psychiatric services. Women with psychiatric disorders can remain with their premature or ill infant, and there is ready liaison with paediatricians for women anxious about their infants.

In-patient admission

The philosophies of units vary. The welfare of mother, infant and family are of primary concern and a holistic approach is probably ideal.

Woman

Individual and group therapy can be structured to meet specific needs as well as covering common themes such as guilt, anger and anxiety. The woman may need time for herself, to deal with her own problems, as well as adapting to her new role. The problem of sleep deprivation often needs to be addressed.

Mother-infant

Assistance, encouragement and support need to be offered. Nursing staff are not there to take over as the infant's mother, except briefly at times of severe distress. They are able to offer support and guidance to help increase the woman's confidence.

Mother-infant groups, looking at infant cues and parental expectations, can help address issues within this developing relationship. Baby massage can be helpful for some women to encourage involvement with their infant.

Partners

In-patient admissions should ideally allow partners and older siblings to be involved. Most units only allow infants under 12 months, but many can have partners stay overnight, and provide the partners with support and counselling. The Mercy Unit offers a fathers' group, run by a male psychiatric nurse, looking at their specific issues. An admission can be a time for reassessment of the relationship and, where primary or secondary problems exist, these can be worked on, to ease the transition home and decrease stress on the woman and her family after discharge.

Transition home

The changes that often need to occur for the family situation to be 'normal' again frequently take considerable time, and admission may only begin and direct such changes. Much can be gained in 4 to 6 weeks (the average Mercy admission), but the situation at home is no longer as it was before this child's birth. The presence of the child back at home will be another change, and the child itself is continuing to develop. Families need to be prepared for this, to know not to expect a 'magic cure', and to learn to adapt to the changes affecting them. Weekend leaves, extended periods at home, returning as a day patient and linking to community supports help this process.

Day patients

Attending hospital as a day patient offers many of the advantages of admission, but with less perceived stigma and disruption to family life. For in-patients it can serve as a transition from hospital to home. Unfortunately, such facilities are limited, and the difficulties of packing up a young infant, the presence of older siblings and the distance required to travel may reduce attendance and thus effectiveness.

Cox's (1991) unit in Stoke-on-Trent, United Kingdom, is independent of an in-patient unit and offers women attendance for 3 to 6 months. They report on the usefulness of this facility, which is linked closely to primary caregivers.

Currently, day-patient facilities at the Mercy are limited to former in-patients.

Specialised home-care services

Oates (1982) offers an alternative to admission—an intensive specialised team able to maintain even severely ill women in their homes, in conjunction with a supportive family. Unfortunately, this is labour-intensive and often perceived as too expensive, but the benefit to women and their families is enormous. Oates reports that although their illnesses did not resolve more quickly than those hospitalised, the women and their partners perceived the time as being shorter. The short-term effects on families were far more beneficial, and longer-term effects may also exist.

Case example – 1

Fatima, a 30-year-old Turkish woman, had strong opposition from her family to the prospect of admission despite a moderate to severe depressive illness. Her husband, although supportive, was sceptical of psychology. There was no one to care for their 2 older children, so while she was in hospital he took unpaid leave. She was forced to discharge herself after 10 days due to a severe financial crisis. There were few supports available in her area; a visiting team, had it been available, could have offered psychological and practical support, and enabled a less stressful recovery period. Fatima's recovery was slow and impeded by financial and family stresses.

Case example – 2

Margerita (see Chapter 9) and her husband had been reluctant for her to be admitted with her first postpartum psychosis. When well, she reiterated that hospitalisation had been a major stress for her. With her subsequent pregnancy, she again experienced a severe postpartum depression with psychotic elements—but before the birth she and her husband had planned that should this occur, she would remain at home. Because of the previous knowledge of her rapid response to treatment, and a supportive motivated family who did 'shifts' at home, Margerita was not hospitalised. She again responded quickly, and she and her husband felt a far greater sense of achievement, maintaining their autonomy and independence, with few negative feelings about the experience.

Community services

Involvement of community services can be an important part of management after discharge, and for out-patients with postpartum psychiatric disorders.

The visit to a doctor or other health professional is a small part of the week, while the illness and the stress of child care is with the woman constantly and a crisis may flare at any time. The woman and her family need to have someone they can contact at any time; if there are regular community contacts the need for such crisis calls is usually diminished.

Crisis line

For some women, knowing they can get help at any time is crucial. It is more likely to be reassuring and of assistance if they are able to call someone specialised in this area than a general crisis line. Such crisis calls are accepted by some general practitioners, support groups, mother-baby units and maternal-child health nurses. Alerting the women in advance as to whom they can ring may prevent the need arising.

Child care services

Many women with postpartum depression burden themselves with the goal of being a 'super mother'. This often, to their mind, means that they must be available for their child or children at all times. Their inability to allow themselves a break accentuates their anxiety; deep-seated resentment breeds anger, guilt and despair.

Part of the treatment can be helping women come to terms with it being acceptable to have someone else care for their child, and that it is unrealistic for them to always be there. Eventually, the child will grow up, go to school, stay with friends. The separation must be faced; its occurrence at a younger age is usually more stressful for the mother than the infant.

The woman needs to be comfortable with the length of time spent away from the infant, and with the caregiver. For some, a family member is the only acceptable alternative to themselves. For others, their mother or mother-in-law is perceived as critical and this in itself is a stress.

Most councils offer a variety of child care services, with fees being means tested. These include crèches, occasional care and family daycare. Nannies are another alternative, and not necessarily more expensive when there is more than one child, but nannies are beyond the scope of many families.

The time-out period need not be long, but it is important to allow the woman to regain her sense of self and to re-adjust to her changed world.

Home help

In keeping with overly high expectations of themselves as mothers, many women with postpartum depression, particularly those with obsessional personalities, expect their houses to be spotless. Others, particularly with psychotic illnesses, may be disorganised and have poor concentration, making basic housework difficult. Home help, assisting with basic household chores, can help alleviate the stress and time commitment needed for these tasks.

Case example

Louise, 28, had 2 children under 4. With the onset of her depression after the second, she felt her life was getting out of control. She felt an overwhelming need to have order around her, but found that even minor tasks were time-consuming and at times impossible. It took her several attempts to make up bottles, as she would forget how much formula she had added, or would realise she had not sterilised the bottles. Home help, assisting her with major tasks, allowed her to devote her time to her children without feeling pressured to attend to less important tasks, and to maintain order in her surroundings.

Family aid

This service is not always readily available, but a family aid in the home for a few hours a day, a number of times a week, can offer practical support and guidance in the short term. This can be particularly useful for women with minimal supports, who have a poor sense of self and who have had a poor role model.

Case example

Rebecca, a 22-year-old mother of 2 who was from an emotionally deprived and physically abusive background, described herself premorbidly as disorganised. A brief psychotic illness, the care of 2 young children—one of whom was epileptic—and a physically abusive partner accentuated this disorganisation. A family aid was able to help her organise a daily routine and to bring some stability to her home environment. This provided a base from which she could work on longer-term issues.

Maternal-child health services

The community maternal-child health (MCH) nurse is a valuable resource for new mothers, particularly ones who, as a function of their psychotic disorder, lack confidence in their mothering skills. Regular contact, with non-judgmental practical guidance, can be a key to surviving the early weeks and months of motherhood. For women who find change difficult, the constantly changing nature of her infant may produce great maternal anxiety—and demand great patience from the maternal-child health nurse.

Such centres can also be the setting for new mothers' groups, which can help some women to achieve a sense of belonging and perspective.

In Australia, the MCH nurse is the one person who sees every new mother. It is he or she who picks up many postpartum depressions; such nurses are one of the major referral sources to the Mercy, to its in-patient unit and out-patient clinic. A recent trial in Melbourne of the Edinburgh Postnatal Depression Scale (Cox 1983) by MCH nurses has recommended its routine use. Certainly, the self-rating scale takes only a few minutes to complete and is highly reliable, having been designed and validated on postnatally depressed women (Harris et al 1989a). It may be particularly useful to introduce it routinely where funding cuts have limited the amount of time MCH nurses are able to spend with women. Scott (1992) put forward a strong argument that the role of the MCH nurse should in fact be increased. It would be a tragedy to lose the valuable training in postpartum disorders and recognition of postpartum disorders being achieved, when it is only in recent years that much of this recognition and referral has occurred.

Support groups

A number of support groups for specific psychiatric disorders exist, usually run wholly or partly by sufferers and ex-sufferers. In Melbourne, a postpartum depression group (PANDA) is a very strong advocate for women with psychiatric illness postpartum. Beside having a substantial political voice, the group has helped increased public awareness and recognition of the disorder. It offers a crisis line, support meetings, educational material and professional speakers. For some women, knowing they are not alone and hearing from ex-sufferers themselves that things can improve can help allay anxiety.

Reading material

Beside useful literature available from self-help groups, 2 books aimed at postnatal depression/psychosis sufferers are available. They are well written and many women and their families find them a useful adjunct to professional help:

- Bryanne Barnett, *Coping with Postnatal Depression*, Lothian, Victoria, 1991; and
- Carol Dix, *The New Mothering Syndrome*, Allen & Unwin, 1987.

CHAPTER 11

The long-term outlook

One of the distinguishing factors about antenatal or postnatal psychiatric illnesses is the presence of the infant. As has been discussed, it is essential to consider the infant in the management of the illnesses. It also has implications in the long term: what happens to these women, and their families, and what is the impact on the child?

The episode—duration and recurrence

The duration of an episode of psychiatric illness occurring in the postpartum period, while needing to be viewed in the light of any previous episodes, may be complicated by the very particular psychosocial stresses at that time. Unlike many other stressors (for instance, financial, grief and so on), the presence of a child is constant. Even when there is child care and support at home, the demands and expectations do not abate. Unlike other jobs, that of a parent is there day and night. One of my patients recently calculated that allowing for her 6 hours of child care a week and the 3 undisturbed nights that she had (on average) a week, she was the responsible caregiver for 3 preschool children for 138 hours a week.

Illnesses such as eating disorders, schizophrenia and bipolar disorder will be at risk of relapse with these stresses, as is true of these illnesses at other times. Non-compliance with medication may be an issue where there is concern about the risk to the infant from drug exposure.

First presentation psychotic and acute-depressive symptoms may respond relatively quickly to medication; psychosocial adjustments take longer. More worrying is the increasing evidence that these episodes may not be as brief and isolated as previously thought. Pitt (1968) found one-third of women were still depressed 1 year later. Uddenberg and Englesson (1978) reported that of 16 women with severe mental illnesses in the postpartum period, half had repeated and/or prolonged problems with their mental health in the following 4 years.

In a follow-up of 15 women with a depressive illness postpartum necessitating admission of 13, and medication in all, 9 women were still on antidepressants 3 to 5 years later (Buist & Janson, in press). Three of these 9 women had had a further child—a fourth had also had a child, but although she required medication was no longer on it. Two women not on medication were clinically depressed.

These findings suggest that for some women motherhood is chronically marred by depression. Uddenberg and Englesson (1978) reported that the group with on-going problems also experienced greater marital disharmony and greater difficulties in the mothering role. It can be speculated that many marital break-ups occurring for some years after the birth of a child may be related to psychiatric illness.

The effect on child development has been documented (Chapter 7). Lee and Gotlib's study (1989) suggested that it is maternal psychopathology, rather than the diagnosis that related to child maladjustment, which implicates a wide variety of maternal psychiatric illnesses. Brevity of episode may not be any reason to be reassured; Coghill et al (1986) and Wrate et al (1985) both found that a brief episode, or episodes occurring particularly in the first year of life, were associated with later cognitive deficits. It may be that this early occurrence of illness permanently disables some mothers by setting a course marked by guilt and feelings of inadequacy. Studies have yet to be conducted to find ways of improving this outcome. Initial studies by Cooper and Murray (1994) have looked at therapeutic techniques with short-term apparent benefits to the mother, but possibly not to the infant. The author's recently completed study (Buist & Janson, in press), although limited by its small size, suggests that children of these women who had high levels of antidepressant in plasma and breast milk, did *better* cognitively. This suggests that aggressive treatment is important.

The clinician must be aware of the possibility of chronicity and its effects, and include this in any management plan.

1. Treat aggressively. Remember that depression postpartum is under-diagnosed, and its severity often not realised. Any medication needs to be of adequate dose. For tricyclics this means over 100 mg/d, often up to 225 mg/d, depending on the experience of side-effects.
2. Treat holistically. Look at psychosocial factors. Remember the partner, infant and older children.
3. Use maximum supports for maximum time.
4. Where possible, without undermining the woman's role, encourage the partner to be involved in playing with and caring for the child.
5. Treat long term. This may mean a longer time period on antidepressants or recommencing at a later time, but also beginning individual, marital, family therapy or parent–infant therapy.

Case example – 1

Sarah, 38, presented initially 12 months postpartum after her first child, Emma, was born. Her general practitioner, after many months of believing her symptoms of anxiety and tearfulness were normal adjustment in a first-time mother, exaggerated because she was an 'elderly primipara', had finally put her on antidepressants a month prior. Sarah appeared a warm and loving mother; she was also very anxious about her own health and her capacity to be a perfect mother. Her husband's loss of job had created financial anxieties, and placed her in a dilemma as she believed it was the mother's role to be at home. With increasing time, the marital friction increased.

Sarah had 12 months of supportive counselling, and her acute symptoms settled. She no longer experienced panic attacks and was rarely tearful. She rated herself as only 60% of her normal self, however.

When Emma was just over 2, Sarah became pregnant again; possibly in part as an act of defiance to indicate to her husband that she wished him to return to work, and also indicating an inability to work in a partnership and put aside her own firm ideas of how many children she wanted. She was also considerably pressured by her age.

The original symptoms returned through pregnancy and worsened postpartum. Her over-protectiveness of Emma heightened, with major difficulties in limit setting. The older child 'breastfed' throughout the pregnancy because of Sarah's fear of saying no. Her husband, although at home, was excluded from a major parenting role. At 3½, Emma had behavioural problems and Sarah continued treatment for a depressive disorder.

Sarah had a chronic low-grade depressive illness, with individual issues, that had a severe impact on her capacity to care for 2 children. There was little support from her husband, but little desire or ability to engage this; the therapist perhaps could have been more encouraging of couple sessions. Mother–child sessions were important to the welfare of both children.

Case example – 2

Laura, 30, presented after the birth of her second child, Jackson, with no past or family psychiatric history. She had worked as a lawyer up until the birth of her first child and had continued some involvement in her husband's law firm until the arrival of her second child.

After the birth of Jackson, Laura suffered a number of physical complaints and had extensive investigations. When these (including a myelogram, CT scan and a vast array of blood tests) were normal, she was referred to a psychiatrist.

Laura presented as an intelligent, pleasant and articulate woman— who didn't feel depressed. She described fatigue, poor concentration, low motivation and difficulties sleeping; in view of the negative medical results, antidepressants were commenced. Her initial response was very good; this, however, settled over time so that at best she was only 70% of her normal self, and frequently only 40%. The major effect was on her ability to entertain or socialise, an important part of her role as wife to a senior partner of a law firm. She also felt totally unable to return to work. This was not an important issue for her husband, who was very supportive, but it was for Laura.

Several changes of medication resulted in major side-effects and deterioration, so Laura was continued on the same medication. After 4 years, she still remained at only 70% (at best) of her usual self. She had wished for a third child, but had decided this was no longer a risk she was prepared to take.

A number of issues are raised in this case. Firstly, Laura was overwhelmed by the duration of her illness. Supportive groups and her treating doctor had encouraged her to believe that she would be better by Jackson's second birthday. She was not by his fourth. This is not so for all women, but practitioners need to be reminded of what *is* the reality for a significant proportion.

Secondly, there is the issue whether alternative medications should have been pursued more vigorously: at 4 years after the onset Laura was willing to try newer drugs that had not previously been on the market. And thirdly, there is the role of psychological therapies. Laura had individual therapy which helped her to link the role that life stresses had had in worsening her symptoms. This aided her in setting limits for herself, something she had previously been unable to do. Over the 4 years, although the fatigue continued, depression largely took over as the predominating symptom.

But although this helped her to deal with her illness, therapy did not cure what appeared to be a biologically-based disorder.

Future pregnancies

Kendell et al (1987) calculated that the postpartum period is the time of highest risk for a woman of having a psychiatric illness. They believed this risk decreased antenatally—but this may reflect the misdiagnosis of psychiatric symptoms as 'normal antenatal anxiety'—and increased 35-fold in the mother, postpartum. They also believed that this risk did not return to normal until 2 years postpartum.

This risk will be highest for women with factors in their history leading them to be prone to psychiatric illness. For women who have had an episode of psychiatric illness postpartum, their risk of a recurrence is higher with any future pregnancy. The degree of risk of recurrence is uncertain and estimates vary. The more severe the illness, pregnancies within 2 years of the child with whom the first illness occurred, associated failure to fully recover, and continued or recurrent psychosocial stresses, are all likely to increase the risk of recurrence.

Women and their partners need to be informed of this risk. Adequate contraception is essential while the woman is ill and/or on medication, and preferably until after the 2 year postpartum period is over. There are teratogenic risks of some medications (see Chapter 8) and a pregnancy occurring while a woman is depressed may worsen the depression and complicate treatment, putting the foetus at risk. Alternatively, some women report their mental state to improve throughout pregnancy; it may then deteriorate postpartum. It is up to the partners to decide how to deal with the risk of, or actual, pregnancy, but informing them early of the risks at least increases their chances of being able to make an informed decision.

For many women, the lowered libido from the combined effects of the low levels of oestrogen and of the depression mean that intercourse is infrequent. For these women, particularly if breastfeeding, condoms may be the preferred contraception. Anecdotally, some women feel the mini-pill worsens their depression. This does not appear true of the other contraceptive pills, but where there is a history of mood disturbance associated with the contraceptive pill, it should be avoided. For some, returning to a form of contraception with which they are confident is important in relieving their fear of conceiving at this time.

Outcomes of subsequent pregnancies can be optimised by:

1. delaying until:
   (a) over 2 years postpartum,
   (b) and fully recovered,
   (c) and off medication for 1 year;
2. consulting a supportive health professional throughout the pregnancy and through the postpartum period. This health professional should themselves be able to treat any psychiatric illness occurring postpartum, or be associated with any such treatment;
3. seeing partners prior to and through the pregnancy;
4. emphasising the supportive and practical, looking to minimise the stresses associated with the birth, for example, partner to take time off work, supportive relative to stay with or care for older children, or be available to do so, not moving house or renovating;
5. commencing lithium or carbamazepine, for those women previously successfully treated with these, soon after delivery if the woman is not breastfeeding. Current studies (Brockington et al, unpublished) are evaluating the effectiveness of such intervention.

Case example – 1

Margerita (see Chapters 9 and 10) had a severe depressive episode after her first child. She had her second child just over 2 years after her first. Again there was a severe psychotic episode; again her symptoms responded quickly to medication without need for hospitalisation and with no apparent effect on her child's development.

Case example – 2

Dale, 25, a postal worker, experienced a severe psychotic episode after the birth of her first child. There was a strong family history of bipolar disorder. She required in-patient treatment for 10 months, including antidepressants, major tranquillisers, lithium and ECT. She had not fully recovered until 2 years postpartum, and remained on medication until 3 years postpartum. At this time, she and her husband consulted me regarding having another child. The decision to do so, or not, had to be theirs; while it is not the clinician's role to advise them, it was important that they be aware of the risks. They spoke to me at length, and at a subsequent appointment they informed me that *any* risk of a recurrence was too great: they were particularly concerned as there was no close family member to care for Dale. They elected not to go through with another pregnancy, but adopted a special needs baby.

Risk factors

A number of researchers have evaluated antenatally risk factors that correlate with subsequent postpartum depression (Dennerstein et al 1989; Kumar & Robson 1984; O'Hara et al 1984; Cox et al 1982). The risk factors include:
1. history of psychiatric illness, particularly a previous postpartum disorder;
2. family history of psychiatric illness, particularly affective disorder;
3. history of childhood sexual abuse;
4. marital difficulties;
5. poor social supports;
6. poor family relationships and support, particularly a poor relationship with mother;
7. history of premenstrual tension;
8. obsessional personality characteristics.

A history of a particular psychiatric disorder may also predispose women to a recurrence (for example, schizophrenia, bipolar disorder). A history of childhood sexual abuse, we know, predisposes women to a variety of psychiatric disorders, and this may be true in the postpartum period but remains to be assessed (Buist & Barnett, in press).

Prevention

Given the identification of risk factors, it is reasonable to assume that many women prone to psychiatric illness postpartum can be identified antenatally.

There is little published research on prevention of postpartum depression or the effects of antenatal education. The final report of the Ministerial Review of Birthing Services in Victoria (1990) noted women's concerns about the birthing process, the high incidence of postpartum depression, and recommended that childbirth education programs incorporate discussion on issues relating to the transition to parenthood. Leverton and Elliott (1988) produced and piloted a questionnaire which showed 40% of women with identified risk factors subsequently developed depression, compared with 16% of controls.

Hillier and Slade (1989) looked at the effects of antenatal classes on women's anxiety and knowledge and concluded that the major gains were in the latter area, and that anxiety was unrelated to knowledge. These anxious women may have been an 'at risk' group which could benefit more from antenatal classes with a different emphasis and structure.

Stewart (1985) noted an increase in women associating postpartum psychiatric illness with the birth experience and felt this was associated with classes run by non-medically qualified staff, and the emphasis of classes on labour itself, rather than the outcome—that is, a live, healthy mother and baby.

Gordon and Gordon (1960) used a psychosocial approach, supporting women antenatally with additional antenatal classes and found these women to subsequently experience less emotional trauma.

Halonen and Passman (1985) looked at the effect of relaxation training antenatally and found this to reduce postpartum distress and to possibly facilitate the mother–infant relationship.

Elliott et al (1988) identified women at risk of postpartum depression and offered these women a supportive group antenatally, and found, when compared to a matched control group, that the incidence of postpartum depression was lowered, particularly in first-time mothers. Her emphasis was on continuity of care, easy access to individual help, support over education, restricted membership and focusing beyond the birth (Elliott 1989). Although these groups included preparation for parenthood, it seems they were not an alternative to antenatal classes—rather, an addition.

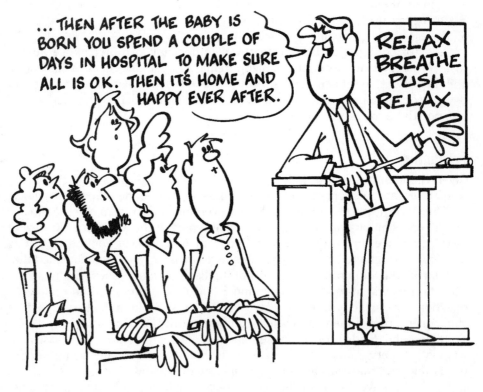

Classes emphasise labour rather than the outcome—a live, healthy mother and baby

There is clearly a need to reduce the incidence of postpartum mood disorders. What little research has been published in this area suggests that antenatal intervention reduces postpartum emotional disturbance and, in particular, postpartum depression. At present antenatal classes do not deal with the issues of motherhood for which many vulnerable women need to prepare themselves.

A change of direction is strongly recommended.

Community services

Australia
ACT
Postnatal Depression Support Group
PO Box 1705, Tuggeranong
Mail Delivery Centre 2901
Queen Elizabeth Home: (06) 248 0813

New South Wales
In-patient/crisis counselling
Karitane: (02) 399 7111
Tresillian: (02) 568 3633
      (02) 958 8931
Tresillian Outreach: (02) 958 3076
       (02) 568 3633
Tresillian Day Clinic: (02) 436 4086

Queensland
In-patient
Mothercraft Home: (07) 252 8555
      (07) 262 4863
New Farm Clinic, New Farm (private): (07) 358 3888
Prince Charles Hospital (Winston Noble Unit): (07) 3350 8111
The Belmont Hospital (private): (07) 398 0111

Support group
Postnatal Distress Support Group: (07) 358 4988

South Australia
In-patient
Glenside Hospital (Helen Mayo House): (08) 303 1111
Torrens House: (08) 236 0453

Support groups
Mothers Support Group: (08) 632 3711
Overcoming Postnatal Disturbance: (08) 268 9330
Postnatal Depression Support Group: (08) 282 1206
Queen Vic Hospital Support Group: (08) 332 4888

Tasmania
In-patient
Mothercraft Home: (002) 30 2700

Victoria
Crisis lines
Post and Antenatal Depression Association (PANDA): (03) 9882 5756
Maternal and Child Health Nurse Crisis Line: (03) 9853 0844

In-patient
Austin Family Unit: (03) 9496 5000
Canterbury Family Centre: (03) 9882 8336
Larundel Mother-Baby Unit: (03) 9280 0289
Mercy Hospital for Women Mother-Baby Unit: (03) 9270 2501
Melbourne Clinic Mother-Baby Unit (private): (03) 9429 4688
Monash Mother-Baby Unit: (03) 9550 2325
Pathway Parent Infant (private): (03) 9833 4644
O'Connell Centre: (03) 9882 2326
Queen Elizabeth Centre: (03) 9347 2777
Tweddle Child and Family Health Service: (03) 9689 1577

Out-patient
Abbacare: (03) 9379 9099
Canterbury Family Centre: (03) 9882 8336
Caroline Chisholm: (03) 9370 3933
Mercy Hospital for Women, Postnatal Disorder Clinic: (03) 9270 2884

Support group
PANDA:
- Administration: (03) 9882 5396
- Support: (03) 9882 5756

Western Australia
Clinics and centres specialising in PPD
Gosnells Women's Health Clinic: (09) 490 2258
Granny Spier's Community Home: (09) 401 2699
Lockridge Community Health and Development Centre: (09) 279 0100
Multicultural Women's Health Centre: (09) 335 8214
Nygala Family Resources Centre: (09) 367 7855

Parent Help Centre: (09) 272 1466
PND Professional Association: (09) 382 0873
Southwell Child Health Services Centre: (09) 418 1177
Wanslea Family Support Service: (09) 384 2600

Crisis lines
Crisis Care: (09) 325 1111
Ngala Family Resource Centre: (09) 367 3256
● Monday to Friday 8.30 am – 10.00 pm
● Weekends and public holidays 8.00 am – 1.00 pm, 5.00 pm – 10.00 pm
Parent Help Centre: (09) 325 1111

Groups
May run at listed centres
Drs M. Jones and G. McKenzie: (09) 381 7111

In-patient
Niola Hospital (private): (09) 381 1833

Canada
Clinic and centre specialising in PPD
Postpartum Adjustment Support Services (PASS-Canada)
Aid for New Mothers
Eileen G. Beltzner, Executive Director
PO Box 7282
Oakville Ont LBJ BCB
Tel: (905) 897 6262

Self-help groups
Calgary Postpartum Support Society (CPSS)
Honey Watts, Executive Director
310–707 Tenth Ave SW
Calgary AL T2R 0B3
Tel: (408) 266 3083

Mothers Offering Mothers Support (MOMS)
PO Box 4001, Station E
Ottawa Ont K IS 5B1

Pacific Post Partum Society (PPPS)
Suite 104/1416 Commercial Drive
Vancouver BC B5L 3X9
Tel: (604) 255 7999

New Zealand
Clinics and centres specialising in PPD
Karitane: (09) 69 8539
  (04) 89 6075
  (03) 66 0765
  (03) 48 9447
Royal New Zealand Plunket Society: (09) 77 4365

Republic of Ireland
Support group
Post-Natal Distress Association of Ireland
Carmichael Centre
North Brunswick St
Dublin 7
Tel: (010531) 872 7172

United Kingdom
Clinic and centre specialising in PPD/PPP
Parent-Child Day Centre
C/- Department of Psychiatry
North Staffordshire Hospital
Thornburrow Dr
Hartshill
Stoke-on-Trent
Tel: (01782) 716 019

International organisation specialising in PPD
Marce Society
Dr Trevor Friedman, Secretary
Department of Psychiatry
Leicester Hospital
Leicester LE5 4PW
Tel: (0116) 249 0490

Support groups
Association for Postnatal Illness
Mrs Clare Delpech
7 Gowan Ave
Fulham London SE 25 4HS UK
Tel: 071 731 4108

Association for Postnatal Illness
25 Jerdan Pl
Fulham London SW6 1BE UK
Tel: (0171) 386 0868

Meet-a-Mum-Association
Briony Hallam
58 Malden Ave
South Norwood London SE 25 4HS UK
Tel: 081 656 7318

Postnatal Illness Support Link
16 Leybourne Ave
Forest Hall
Newcastle Upon Tyne NE12 OAP UK

Premenstrual Syndrome and Postnatal Depression Support
C/- 113 University St
Belfast N Ireland BT7 1HP UK
Tel: (01232) 653 209

United States

Clinics and centres specialising in PPD/PPP

Cass House Women's Center
Joan Woodle, MD
133 Quaker Path Road
East Setauket NY 11733
Tel: (516) 689 5664

Center for Postpartum Depression
Joyce A. Venis, RNC
33 Witherspoon St
Princeton NJ 08540
Tel: (609) 497 1144

Duke Postpartum Support Program
William S. Meyers, MSW, BCD
Duke University Medical Center
PO Box 3812
Durham NC 27710
Tel: (919) 684 3714

Barbara Lewin, MD
2400 Chestnut Street, Suite 2203
Philadelphia PA 19103
Tel: (215) 561 6381

Mother Matters
Regional Center for Mother and Child Care at Memorial Hospital
615 North Michigan St
South Bend IN 46601
Tel: (219) 284 3456

Postpartum Mood Disorders Clinic
Susan Hickman, PhD
Robert Hickman, PhD
6635 Crawford St
San Diego CA 92129
Tel: (619) 287 2442

Postpartum Stress Centre
Rosemount Plaza
1062 Lancaster Ave
Rosemount PA 19010

Pregnancy and Postpartum Treatment Program
Valerie Raskin, MD
Laura Miller, MD
University of Illinois
912 South Wood St
Chicago IL 60612
Tel: (312) 996 2972

Self-help groups

Depression After Deliver (DAD)
PO Box 1282
Morrisville PA 19067
Tel: (215) 295 3994

PAM (Postpartum Assistance for Mothers)
PAM East Bay
PO Box 20515
Castro Valley CA 95633
Tel: (810) 727 4610 (Shoshana)

PAM South Bay
15100 Lynn Ave
Los Gatos CA 95032
Tel: (415) 948 8053 (Diana)
(408) 356 7872

The Emotional You
Santa Barbara Birth Resource Centre
1525 Santa Barbara St
Santa Barbara CA 93101
Tel: (805) 966 4545

Support groups

Postpartum Health Alliance
PO Box 341 280
Los Angeles CA 90034
Tel: (310) 915 7028

Postpartum Support, International (PSI)
Jane Honikman, Founder
927 North Kellogg Ave
Santa Barbara CA 83111
Tel: (805) 967 7636

Bibliography

Aftimos, S. (1986). Tobacco, alcohol and marijuana in pregnancy. *Current Therapeutics*; June 29–31.

Ainsworth, M. (1971). Individual differences in strange situation behaviour of one year olds. In: Schaffer, H. R. (ed.). *The Origins of Human Social Relations*. London: Academic Press.

Ainsworth, M. (1975). Social development in the first year of life: maternal influences on infant–mother attachment. Sir Geoffrey Vickers Lecture.

Alanen, Y. O., Kinnunen, P. (1975). Marriage and the development of schizophrenia. *Psychiatry*; 38:346–65.

Alder, E. M. et al (1986). Hormones, mood and sexuality in lactating women. *British Journal of Psychiatry*; 148:74–9.

Alder, E. M., Bancroft, J. (1988). The relationship between breastfeeding persistence, sexuality and mood in postpartum women. *Psychological Medicine*; 18:389–96.

Alder, E. M., Cox, J. L. (1983). Breastfeeding and postnatal depression. *Journal of Psychosomatic Research*; 2739–44.

Alroomi, L. G. et al (1988). Maternal narcotic abuse and the newborn. *Archives of Disease in Childhood*; 63:81–3.

Ananth, J. (1975). Congenital malformations with psychopharmacologic agents. *Comprehensive Psychiatry*; 16:437–45.

Aneshensel, C., Stone, J. (1982). Stress and depression. *Archives of General Psychiatry*; 39:1392–6.

Arana, G. et al (1977). Prolactin levels in milk in depression. *Psychosomatic Medicine*; 39:193–7.

Ayd, F. J. (1968). Phenothiazine therapy during pregnancy: effects on the newborn infant. *Intensive Drug Therapy Newsletter*; 3:39–48.

Ballard, C. G. et al (1994). Prevalence of postnatal psychiatric morbidity in mothers and fathers. *British Journal of Psychiatry*; 164:782–8.

Barclay, L. (1994). Unpublished study 1994. University of Technology, Centre for Graduate Nursing Studies, NSW.

Bardon, D. et al (1968). Mother-baby unit; psychiatric survey of 115 cases. *British Medical Journal*; 5607:755–8.

Barrison, I. G., Waterson, E. J., Murray-Lyon, I. M. (1985). Adverse effects of alcohol in pregnancy. *British Journal of Addiction*; 80:11–22.

Beary, M. D., Merry, J. (1986). The rise in alcoholism in women of fertile age (letter). *British Journal of Addiction*; 81 (1):142.

Beitchman, J. et al (1992). A review of the long term effects of child sexual abuse. *Child Abuse and Neglect*; 16:101–18.

Bielski, R., Friedel, R. O. (1976). Prediction of tricyclic antidepressant response. *Archives of General Psychiatry*; 33:1479–89.

Bifulco, A., Brown, G., Adler, Z. (1991). Early sexual abuse and clinical depression in adult life. *British Journal of Psychiatry*; 159:115–22.

Bion, W. R. (1962). *Learning from Experience.* London: Heinemann.

Birtchnell, J., Kennard, J. (1983). Marriage and mental illness. *British Journal of Psychiatry*; 142:193–8.

Bleuler, E. (1911). *Dementia praecox or the Group of Schizophrenia.* New York: International University Press.

Bowlby, J. (1969). *Attachment and Loss* I. Attachment. London: Hogarth.

Boyce, P. et al (1991). Personality as a vulnerability factor to depression. *British Journal of Psychiatry*; 159:106–14.

Brandon, S. (1982). Depression after childbirth. *British Medical Journal*; 613–14.

Brazelton, T., Cramer, B. (1991). *The Earliest Relationship.* Karnac Books.

Breier, A., Strauss, J. (1984). The role of social relationships in recovery from psychotic disorders. *American Journal of Psychiatry*; 141(8):949–55.

Brezinka, C. et al (1994). Denial of pregnancy: obstetrical aspects. *Journal of Psychosomatic Obstetrics and Gynaecology*; 15:35–43.

Brinch, M., Isager, T., Tolstrip, K. (1988). Anorexia nervosa and motherhood: reproduction pattern and mothering behaviour of 50 women. *Acta Psychiatrica Scandinavia*; 77:611–17.

Brockington, I. F. et al (1981). Puerperal psychosis, phenomena and diagnosis. *Archives of General Psychiatry*; 38:829–33.

Brockington, I. F., Cox-Roper, A. (1982). Nosology of puerperal mental illness. In: Brockington, I. F., Kumar, R. (eds). *Motherhood and Mental Illness.* UK: Buttermouth, 1–16.

Brody, G., Forehand, R. (1986). Maternal perceptions of child maladjustment as a function of the combined influence of child behaviour and maternal depression. *Journal of Consulting Clinical Psychology*; 54 (2):237–40.

Brown, G. W., Harris, T. (1978). *The Social Origin of Depression.* London: Tavistock.

Brown, M. (1986). Marital support during pregnancy. *Journal of Obstetric and Gynaecological Nursing*; 475–83.

Bryer, B., Nelson, B. A., Krol, P. A. (1987). Childhood sexual and physical abuse as factors in adult psychiatric illness. *American Journal of Psychiatry*; 144:1426–36.

Buist, A. (1994). Heresy, hormones and husbands: a hypothetical case of postpartum depression. *Australasian Psychiatry*; 2 (4):185.

Buist, A., Barnett, B. Childhood sexual abuse—a risk factor for postpartum depression? (Accepted by *Australian and New Zealand Journal of Psychiatry*; 1995.)

Buist, A., Janson, H. The effect of exposure to dothiepin and northiaden in breast milk on child development. (Accepted by *British Journal of Psychiatry*; 1995.)

Buist, A., Norman, T., Dennerstein, L. (1990). Breastfeeding and the use of psychotropic medication. *Journal of Affective Disorders*; 19:197.

Buist, A., Norman, T., Dennerstein, L. (1993). Plasma and breast milk concentrations of dothiepin and northiaden in lactating women. *Human Psychopharmacology*; 8:29–33.

Bundrock, V. (1989). Australian breastfeeding statistics. *Nursing Mothers' Association of Australia Newsletter*; 5:3–6.

Burkett, L. (1991). Parenting behaviours of women who were sexually abused as children in their families of origin. *Family Process*; 30:421–34.

Caplan, H. L. et al (1989). Maternal depression and the emotional development of the child. *British Journal of Psychiatry*; 154:818–22.

Carroll, B. (1972). The hypothalmic-pituitary adrenal axis in depressive illness. In: Dansi (ed.). *Depressive Illness—Some Research Studies.* Springfield, Illinois.

Carroll, J. (1977). The intergenerational transmission of family violence. *Aggressive Behaviour*; 3:289–99.

Coghill, S. R. et al (1986). Impact of maternal depression in cognitive development of young children. *British Medical Journal*; 292:1165–7.

Cohler, B. et al (1980). Child care attitudes and development of young children of mentally ill and well mothers. *Psychological Reports*; 46:31–46.

Cole, P. et al (1992). Parenting difficulties among adult survivors of father–daughter incest. *Child Abuse and Neglect*; 16:239–49.

Cole, P., Woolger, C. (1989). Incest survivors: the relation of their perception of their parents and their own parenting behaviour. *Child Abuse and Neglect*; 13:409–16.

Condon, J. T., Hilton, C. A. (1988). A comparison of smoking and drinking behaviour in pregnancy: who abstains and why. *Medical Journal of Australia*; 148 (8):381–5.

Condon, J. T., Watson, T. L. (1987). The maternity blues: exploration of psychological hypotheses. *Acta Psychiatrica Scandinavia*; 76:164–71.

Cooper, P., Murray, L. (1994). Three psychological treatments for postnatal depression: a controlled comparison. Marce Society Conference, Cambridge, UK, September.

Cooper, P. J. et al (1988). Nonpsychotic psychiatric disorder after childbirth. *British Journal of Psychiatry*; 152:799–806.

Cox, A. et al (1987). The impact of maternal depression in young children. *Journal of Child Psychology and Psychiatry*; 28 (6):917–28.

Cox, J. (1983). Clinical and research aspects of postnatal depression. *Journal of Psychosomatic Obstetrics and Gynaecology*; 2–1:46–52.

Cox, J. (1991). Postnatal depression in the potteries. Marce Society Conference, London, July.

Cox, J., Connor, Y., Kendell, R. E. (1982). Prospective study of psychological disorders of childbirth. *British Journal of Psychiatry*; 140:111–17.

Cox, J., Holden, J., Sagovsky, R. (1987). Detection of postnatal depression: development of 101 item postnatal depression scale. *British Journal of Psychiatry*; 150:782–6.

Cox, J. L. (1988). The life event of childbirth: sociocultural aspects of postnatal depression. In: Kumar, R., Brockington, I. F. (eds). *Motherhood and Mental Illness* 2. London: Wright.

Crepman, J. et al (1985). Concerns of breastfeeding mothers from birth to 4 months. *Nursing Research*; 34:374–7.

Critchley, H. O. D. et al (1988). Fetal death in cocaine abuse. Case Report. *British Journal of Obstetrics and Gynaecology*; 9 (2):195–6.

Crombie, D. L., Pinsert, R. J., Fleming, D. M. (1975). Fetal effects of tranquillisers in pregnancy. *New England Journal of Medicine*; 293:198–9.

Cunningham, A. (1981). Breastfeeding and morbidity in industrialized countries: an update. In: Jeliffer, D. and E. (eds). *Advances in International Maternal Child Health*. New York: Oxford University Press, 128.

Cutrona, C. E. (1982). Non-psychotic postpartum depression: a review of recent research. *Clinical Psychology*; 2:487–503.

Czeizel, A. E., Bod, M., Malasz, P. (1992). *European Journal of Epidemiology*; 8: 122–7.

Dalton, K. (1983). Prophylactic progesterone treatment for postnatal depression. *Marce Society Annual*. London: Marce Society.

Dean, C. and Kendell, R. E. (1981). Symptomatology of puerperal illness. *British Journal of Psychiatry*; 134:128–33.

Dennerstein, L., Lehert, P., Riphagen, F. (1989). Postpartum depression—risk factors. *Journal of Psychosomatic Obstetrics and Gynaecology Supplement*; 10:53–65.

Diagnostic and Statistical Manual of Mental Disorder—DSM IV (1994). Washington: American Psychiatric Association.

Dominion, A. J. (1979). Marriage and psychiatric illness. *British Medical Journal*; 854–5.

Edlund, M. J., Craig, T. J. (1984). Antipsychotic drug use and birth defects: an epidemiologic reassessment. *Comprehensive Psychiatry*; 25:32–7.

Eliahov, H. E. et al (1978). *British Journal of Obstetrics and Gynaecology*; 85: 431–8.

Elliott, S. A. (1989). Psychological strategies in the prevention and treatment of postnatal depression. *Ballieres Clinical Obstetrics and Gynaecology*; 3 (4): 879–903.

Elliott, S. A., Sanjack, M., Leverton, T. (1988). Parent groups in pregnancy. In: Gottlieb, B. H. (ed.). *Marshalling Social Supports. Formats, Processes and Effects*. Beverley Hills, CA: Sage, 87–110.

Emery, R., Weintraub, S., Neale, J. (1982). Effects of mental discord in the school behaviour of schizophrenics, affectively disordered and normal patients. *Journal of Abnormal Child Psychology*; 10:215–28.

Erkkola, R., Kanto, J. (1972). Diazepam and breastfeeding. *Lancet*; 1:1235–6.

Feldman, L. B., Grodman, J., Behrman, D. (1984). Psychiatric symptoms of mentally distressed wives and husbands. 140–5.

Ferry, B., Smith, D. P. (1983). Breastfeeding Differentials Comparison Studies, International Statistical Institute and World Fertility Survey.

Fischman, S. H. et al (1986). Changes in sexual relationships in postpartum couples. *Journal of Obstetric and Gynaecological Nursing*; Jan/Feb: 58–63.

Fisher, J., Stanley, R., Burrows, G. (1990). Psychological adjustment to caesarean childbirth; Psychosom, a review of the evidence. *Obstetrics and Gynaecology*; 11:91–106.

Ford, K., Labhok, M. (1990). Who is breastfeeding? Implications of associated sociological and biomedical variables for research in the consequence of methods of infant feeding. *American Journal of Clinical Nutrition*; 52:451–6.

Fowler, D. B., Brandon, R. E. (1965). A psychiatric mother and baby unit. *Lancet*; 16 January: 160–1.

Fowler, R. C., Tsuang, M. T. (1975). Spouses of schizophrenics. A blind comparative study. *Comprehensive Psychiatry*; 16:334–42.

Fraiberg, S., Adelson, E., Shapiro, V. (1980). Ghosts in the nursery. In: *Clinical Studies in Infant Mental Health.* London: Tavistock.

Gard, D. et al (1986). A multivariate investigation of postpartum mood disturbances. *British Journal of Psychiatry*; 148:567–75.

Gardner, D. K., Rayburn, W. F. (1980). Drugs in breastmilk. In: Rayburn, W. F., Zuspan, F. P. (eds). *Drug Therapy in Obstetrics and Gynacology.* Norfolk, Connecticut: Appleton Century Crofts, 175–96.

Ghodsian, M., Lajicell, E., Wolkend, S. (1984). A longitudinal study of maternal depression and childhood behavioural problems. *Journal of Child Psychology*; 25:91–109.

Gitlin, M., Pasnau, R. (1989). Psychiatric syndromes linked to reproductive function in women: a review of current knowledge. *American Journal of Psychiatry*; 146 (11):1413–22.

Glaser, Y. (1962). A unit of mothers and babies in a psychiatric hospital. *Journal of Child Psychology and Psychiatry*; 53–60.

Goering, P., Lancee, W., Freeman, S. (1992). Marital support and recovery from depression. *British Journal of Psychiatry*; 160:76–82.

Goldberg, H. L., Di Mascio, A. (1978). Psychotropic drugs in pregnancy. In: Lipton, M.A., Di Mascio, A., Killan, K.F. (eds). *Psychopharmacology: A Generation of Progress.* New York: Raven Press, 1047–55.

Goldstein, D. J., Williams, M. L., (1992). *Clinical Research*; 40:168A.

Gordon, R., Kapostins, E., Gordon, K. (1965). Factors in postpartum emotional adjustment. *Obstetrics and Gynaecology*; 25 (2):158–66.

Gordon, R. E., Gordon, K. K. (1960). Social factors in prevention of postpartum emotional problems. *Obstetrics and Gynaecology*; 15 (4):433–8.

Grossman, F., Eichler, L., Winickoft, S. (1980). Pregnancy, birth and parenthood: adaption of mothers, fathers and infants. Jossey Bass.

Halonen, J. S., Passman, R. H. (1985). Relaxation training and expectation in the treatment of postpartum depression. *Journal of Consulting Clinical Psychology*; 53 (6):839–45.

Hamilton, M. (1967). Development of a rating scale for primary depressive illness. *British Journal of Social and Clinical Psychology*; 278–96.

Handley, S. L. et al (1980). Tryptophan, cortisol and puerperal mood. *British Journal of Psychiatry*; 136:498–508.

Hapgood, C., Elkind, G., Wright, J. (1988). Maternity blues: phenomena and relationship to late postpartum depression. *Australian and New Zealand Journal of Psychiatry*; 22:299–306.

Harding, J. (1989). Postpartum disorders: a review. *Comprehensive Psychiatry*, January/February; 30 (1):109–12.

Harris, B. et al (1989a). The use of rating scales to identify postnatal depression. *British Journal of Psychiatry*; 154:813–17.

Harris, B. et al (1989b). The hormonal environment of postnatal depression. *British Journal of Psychiatry*; 154:660–7.

Harris, B. et al (1992). Association between postpartum thyroid dysfunction and thyroid antibodies and depression. *British Medical Journal*; 305:152–6.

Harvey, I., McGrath, G. (1988). Psychiatric morbidity in spouses of women admitted to a mother-baby unit. *British Journal of Psychiatry*; 152:506–10.

Haseltine, F. et al (1985). Psychological interviews in screening couples undergoing in vitro fertilization. *New York Academy of Science*; 442:504–22.

Health Department of Victoria Ministerial Review (1990). Having a baby.

Heinonen, O. P., Slone, D., Shapior, S. (1977). *Birth Defects and Drugs in Pregnancy.* Littleton: Publishing Sciences Group.

Henderson, A. F. et al (1991). Treatment of severe postnatal depression with oestradiol subcutaneous patches. *British Journal of Psychiatry*; 38:816–17.

Henderson, S. (1981). Social relationships, adversity and neuroses: an analysis of prospective observations. *British Journal of Psychiatry*; 138:391–8.

Hill, R. M., Desmond, M. M., Key, J. L. (1966). Extrapyramidal dysfunction in an infant of a schizophrenic mother. *Journal of Pediatrics*; 69:589–95.

Hillier, C. A., Slade, P. (1989). The impact of antenatal classes on knowledge, anxiety and confidence in primiparous women. *Journal of Reproduction Infant Psychology*; 7:3–13.

Hobbs, D. (1965). Parenthood as crisis: a third study. *Journal of Marriage and the Family*; 372–6.

Hopkins, J. (1990). The observed infant of attachment theory. *British Journal of Psychotherapy*; 6:460–74.

Hopkins, J., Marcus, M., Campbell, S. B. (1984). Postpartum depression: a critical review. *Psychological Bulletin*; 95:498–515.

Hyde, N. (1984). Long term effects of childhood sexual abuse. *British Medical Journal*; 26:448–50.

Idanpaan-Heikkla, J., Saxen, L. (1973). Possible teratogenicity of imipramine-chloropyramine. *Lancet*; 2:282–4.

International Classification of Diseases ICD 10 (1992). World Health Organisation, Geneva.

Jacobson, S. J. et al (1992). Prospective multicentre study of pregnancy outcome after lithium exposure during first trimester. *Lancet*; 339:530–3.

Janson, H. (1993). Maternal depression and development in early childhood. Masters Thesis, Faculty of Science, University of Melbourne.

John, A., Mattarel, R. (1989). Incidence and duration of breastfeeding in Mexican-American infants 1970–1982. *American Journal of Clinical Nutrition*; October, 50 (4):868–74.

Jones, K. et al (1991). *New England Journal of Medicine*; 320:1661–6.

Jones, K. L., Smith, D. W. (1973). Recognition of fetal alcohol syndrome in infancy. *Lancet*; 3 November, 995–1001.

Judd, L. L. et al (1982). Blunted prolactin response. *Archives of General Psychiatry*; 39:1413–14.

Kalucy, R. S., Crisp, A. H., Harding, B. (1977). A study of 56 families with anorexia nervosa. *British Journal of Medical Psychology*; 50:381–95.

Kearney, M., Cronenwett, L., Barrett, J. (1990). Breastfeeding problems in the first week postpartum. *Nursing Research*; 39 (2):90–5.

Keller, M. et al (1982). Relapse in major depressive disorder: analysis with the life table. *Archives of General Psychiatry*; August, 39 (8):911–15.

Kelly, P. (1976). The relation of infant temperament and mother's psychopathology to interaction in early injury. In: Reigel, K. F., Meachearn, J. A. (eds). *The Developing Individual in a Changing World*; (1):644–75.

Kendell, R. E. (1985). Emotional factors and physical factors in the genesis of puerperal mental disorders. *Journal of Psychosomatic Research*; 29:3–11.

Kendell, R. E. et al (1981). Mood changes in the first three weeks after childbirth. *Journal of Affective Disorders*; 3:317–26.

Kendell, R. E., Chalmers, J. C., Platz, C. (1987). Epidemiology of puerperal psychosis. *British Journal of Psychiatry*; 150:662–73.

Kendell, R. E., Wainwright, S., Hailey, D. (1976). Influence of childbirth on psychiatric morbidity. *Psychological Medicine*; 6:297–302.

Kennerley, H., Gath, D. (1986). Maternity blues reassessed. *Psychiatric Developments*; 1:1–17.

Kissane, D., Ball, J. R. B. (1988). Postnatal depression and psychosis—a mother and baby unit in a general hospital. *Australian and New Zealand Journal of Obstetrics and Gynaecology*; 28:208–12.

Klaiber, E. L., Braverman, D. M., Vogel, W. (1979). Oestrogen therapy for severe persistent depressions in women. *Archives of General Psychiatry*; 36:550–4.

Klaus, M. H., Kennell, J. H. (1975). *Maternal Infant Bonding*. St. Louis: Mosby & Co.

Klein, D., Depue, R. A. (1985). Obsessional personality traits and risk for bipolar affective disorder: an offspring study. *Journal of Abnormal Psychology*; 95:291–7.

Klenka, H. M. (1986). Babies born in a district general hospital to mothers taking heroin. *British Medical Journal*; 293 (6549):745.

Kline, J. et al (1980). Drinking during pregnancy and spontaneous abortion. *Lancet*; ii:176–80.

Knowles, J. A. (1965). Excretion of drugs in milk—a review. *Journal of Pediatrics*; 66:1068–982.

Kocturk, T., Zetterstrom, R. (1988). Breastfeeding and its promotion. *Acta Paediatrica Scandinavia*; 77:183–90.

Kraeplin, L. (1913). *Lectures on Clinical Psychiatry.* Bailliere, Tindall and Cassey Lenan.

Kuenssberg, E. V., Knox, J. D. (1972). Imipramine in pregnancy. *British Medical Journal*; 2:292.

Kumar, R., Robson, K. (1984). A prospective study of emotional disorder in childbearing women. *British Journal of Psychiatry*; 144:35–47.

Kwok, P. et al (1983). Smoking and alcohol consumption during pregnancy: an epidemiological study in Tasmania. *Medical Journal of Australia*; 1:220–3.

Laegreid, L. et al (1975). Abnormalities in children exposed to benzodiazepan in utero (letter). *Lancet*; 2:498.

Lee, C., Gotlib, I. (1989). Maternal depression and child adjustment: a longitudinal analysis. *Journal of Abnormal Psychology*; 98 (1):78–95.

Leverton, T. J., Elliott, S. A. (1988). Antenatal intervention for postnatal depression. In: Van Hall, E., Evergerd, W. (eds). *The Free Woman.* Carnforth, UK: Parthenon Publishing, 479–86.

Lidz, T. (1958). Schizophrenia and the family. *Psychiatry*; 21:21.

Linden, S., Rich, C. (1983). The use of lithium during pregnancy and lactation. *Journal of Clinical Psychiatry*; 44 (10):358–61.

Lindsay, J. S. B. (1975). Puerperal psychosis: a follow up study of a joint mother and baby treatment programme. *Australian and New Zealand Journal of Psychiatry*; 9:73–6.

Litmen, G. (1986). Women and alcohol problems: finding the questions. *British Journal of Addiction*; 81:60–3.

Lovestone, S., Kumar, R. (1994). Postnatal psychiatric illness: the impact on partners. *British Journal of Psychiatry*; 163:210–16.

Lowe, T. (1990). Breastfeeding: attitudes and knowledge of health professionals. *Australian Family Physician*; 19 March, (3):392–8.

MacGregor, S. N. et al (1987). Cocaine use during pregnancy: adverse prenatal effects. *American Journal of Obstetrics and Gynecology*; September, 157 (3):686–90.

Macintyre, M. (1992). An anthropological view. In: Carter, J. (ed.). *Postnatal Depression: Towards a Research Agenda for Human Services and Health.* Canberra: Looking Glass Press, 11–17.

Main, T. (1985). Mothers and children in psychiatric hospital. *Lancet*; 11:845.

Matheson, I., Lunde, P. K. M., Bredesen, J. E. (1990). Midazolam and nitrazepam in the maternity ward; milk concentrations and clinical effects. *British Journal of Clinical Pharmacology*; 30:787–93.

Matheson, I., Panele, H., Alertsen, A. R. (1985). Respiratory depression caused by N-desmethyldoxepin in breastmilk. *Lancet*; 1124.

Matheson, I., Skujaeraasen, J. (1983). Milk concentrations of flupenthizol, nortriplyline and zvalopenthixol and breast differences between 2 patients. *European Journal of Clinical Pharmacology*; 35:217–20.

McNeil, T. F., Kaij, L., Malmquist-Larsson, A. (1984). Women with nonorganic psychosis: factors associated with pregnancy: effect on mental health. *Acta Psychiatrica Scandinavia*; 70 (3):209–19.

Meares, R., Grimwade, J., Wood, C. (1976). A possible relationship between anxiety in pregnancy and puerperal depression. *Journal of Psychosomatic Research*; 20 (6):605–10.

Meltzer, E. S., Kumar, R. (1985). Puerperal mental illness: clinical features and classification—a study of 142 mother-baby admissions. *British Journal of Psychiatry*; 147:647–54.

Mendlewicz, J. et al (1980). The 24 hour profile of prolactin in depression. *Life Science*; 27:2015–24.

Merikangas, K. (1984). Divorce and assortative mating for depression. *American Journal of Psychiatry*; 141:74–5.

Merikangas, K. et al (1985). Marital adjustment and major depression. *Journal of Affective Disorders*; (9):5–11.

Milkovich, L., Van den Berg, B. J. (1976). An evaluation of the teratogenicity of certain antinauseant drugs. *American Journal of Obstetrics and Gynecology*; 125:244–8.

Mills, M., Meadows, S. (1987). Children of depressed mothers: a follow up at age 5. Report of the British Psychological Society Development Section, September, York.

Mitchell, E. K., Davis, J. H. (1984). Spontaneous births into toilets. *Journal of Forensic Science*; 29:591–6.

Morse, C., Dennerstein, L. (1985). Infertile couples entering an in vitro fertilization programme: a preliminary survey. *Journal of Psychosomatic Obstetrics and Gynaecology*; 4:207–19.

Mortola, J. (1989). The use of psychotropic agents in pregnancy and lactation. *Psychiatric Clinics North America*; 12 March, 1:69–87.

Msuya, J. et al (1990). The extent of breastfeeding in Dunedin 1974–1983. *New Zealand Medical Journal*; 28 February: 68–70.

Mullen, P. et al (1988). Impact of sexual and physical abuse on women's mental health. *Lancet*; 841–5.

Mullen, P. et al (1993). Childhood sexual abuse and mental health in adult life. *British Journal of Psychiatry*; 163:721–32.

Murray, L. (1989). Winnicott and the development psychology of infancy. *British Journal Psychotherapy*; 5 (3).

Oats, J. N. et al (1984). The outcome of pregnancies complicated by narcotic drug addiction. *Australian and New Zealand Journal of Obstetrics and Gynaecology*; 24:14–16.

Oates, M. (1982). The development of an integrated community orientated service for severe postnatal depressive. In: Brockington, I. F., Kumar, R. (eds). *Motherhood and Mental Illness* 2. UK: Buttermouth, 223–38.

O'Brien, T. (1974). Excretion of drugs in human milk. *American Journal of Hospital Pharmacology*; 31:844–54.

O'Connor, M., Johnson, G. H., James, D. I. (1981). Intrauterine effect of phenothiazines. *Medical Journal of Australia*; 1:416–17.

O'Hara, M., Zekoski, E. (1988). Postpartum depression: a comprehensive review. In: Brockington, I. F., Kumar, R. (eds). *Motherhood and Mental Illness* 2. UK: Buttermouth, 17–63.

O'Hara, M. W. (1986). Social support, life events and depression during pregnancy and the postpartum. *Archives of General Psychiatry*; 43:569–73.

O'Hara, M. W. (1987). Postpartum blues, depression and psychosis: a review. *Journal of Psychosomatic Obstetrics and Gynaecology*; 7:205–27.

O'Hara, M. W., Neunaber, D. J., Zekoski, E. M. (1984). Prospective study of postpartum depression: prevalence, course and predictive factors. *Journal of Abnormal Psychology*; 93 (2):158–71.

Oppenheim, G. B. (1983). Postnatal illness and its management. *Journal of Psychosomatic Obstetrics and Gynaecology*; 2–1:40–5.

Paffenberger, R. S. (1964). Epidemiological aspects of postpartum mental illness. *British Journal of Preventative Social Medicine*; 18:189–95.

Paffenberger, R. S. Jr (1982). Epidemiologic aspects of mental illness associated with childbearing. In: Brockington, I. F., Kumar, R. (eds). *Motherhood and Mental Illness* 2. UK: Buttermouth, 19–36.

Palmer, R. L et al (1993). Childhood sexual experiences of adults. A comparison of reports by women psychiatric patients and general practice attenders. *British Journal of Psychiatry*; 163:499–504.

Parker, G. (1979). Parental characteristics in relation to depressive disorders. *British Journal of Psychiatry*; 134:134–8.

Parnas, J., Jorgensen, A. (1987). Characteristics of maternal schizophrenia: impact on diagnostic outcome in children.

Parnas, J. (1988). Assortative mating in schizophrenia: results from the Copenhagen high risk study. *Psychiatry*; 51:56–64.

Pasker-de Jong, P. C. M. et al. (1992). *Acta Obstetrics and Gynaecology Scandinavia*; 71:492–3.

Pastusak, A. et al (1993). Pregnancy outcome following first trimester exposure to fluoxetine. *Journal of the American Medical Association*; 269 (17): 2246–8.

Pauleikhoff, B. (1987). Postpartum major depressive illness. *Marce Society Bulletin*; Summer, 43–7.

Paykel, E. et al (1980). Life events and social support in puerperal depression. *British Journal of Psychiatry*; 136–46.

Paykel, E., Weissman, M. (1973). Social adjustment and depression. *Archives of General Psychiatry*; 28:659–63.

Pitt, B. (1968). Atypical depression following childbirth. *British Journal of Psychiatry*; 114:1325–35.

Pitt, B. (1973). Maternity blues. *British Journal of Psychiatry*; 22:431–3.

Platz, C., Kendell, R. E. (1988). Matched control follow up and family study of puerperal psychosis. *British Journal of Psychiatry*; 153:90–4.

Prothoroe, C. (1969). Puerperal psychosis: a long term study 1927–1961. *British Journal of Psychiatry*; 11 (518):9–30.

Puckering, C. (1989). Annotation: maternal depression. *Journal of Child Psychology and Psychiatry*; 30 (6):807–17.

Quinton, D., Rutter, M. (1985). Family pathology and child psychiatric disorders: a four year perspective study. In: *Longitudinal Studies in Child Psychology and Psychiatry*. Chichester: John Wiley, 91–134.

Reich, T., Winokur, G. (1970). Postpartum psychosis in patients with manic depressive disease. *Journal of Nervous Mental Disorders*; 151:60–8.

Rice, P. L., Ly, B., Lumley, J. (1994). Childbirth and soul loss: the case of a Hmong woman. *Medical Journal of Australia*; 160:577–8.

Richman, N., Stevens, J., Graham, P. (1982). *Preschool to School: A Behavioural Study*. London: New York Academic Press.

Robinson, G. E., Stewart, D. E. (1986). Postpartum disorders. *Canadian Medical Association Journal*; 134:31–7.

Rogosch, F., Mowbray, C., Bogat, A. (1992). Determinants of parenting attitudes in mothers with severe psychopathology. *Development Psychopathology*; (4):469–87.

Rohner, R., Rohner, E. (1980). Antecedents and consequences of parental rejection: a theory of emotional abuse. *Child Abuse and Neglect*; 4:189–98.

Rosa, F. W. (1991). *New England Journal of Medicine*; 324:674–7.

Rosett, H. L., Weiner, L. (1981). Identifying pregnant patients at risk from alcohol. *Canadian Medical Association Journal*; 15 July, 125:149–54.

Rubin, P. C. et al (1986). Prospective survey of use of therapeutic drugs, alcohol, and cigarettes during pregnancy. *British Medical Journal*; 292:81–3.

Rumeau-Roquette, C., Goujard, J., Huel, C. (1977). Possible teratogenic effects of phenothiazines in human beings. *Teratology*; 15 (1):57–64.

Rutter, M., Quinton, D. (1984). Parental psychiatric disorder: effect on children. *Psychological Medicine*; 14:853–80.

Saffra, M. D., Oakley, G. D. (1975). Association between cleft lip with or without cleft palate and prenatal exposure to diazepam. *Lancet*; 2:478–540.

Sameroff, A. J., Seifer, R., Zax, M. (1982). Early development of children at risk for emotional disorders. Masographic of the Society for Research in Development; 47 (7):199.

Schou, M., Amdisen, A. (1973). Lithium and pregnancy III. Lithium ingestion by children breastfed by women on lithium treatment. *British Medical Journal*; 2:138.

Schou, M., Vestergaard, P. (1983). Lithium treatment: problems and precautions. In: Burrows, G. D., Norman, T. R., Davies, B. (eds). *Antidepressants. Drugs in Psychiatry* Vol. 1. Amsterdam: Elsevier Science Publishers, 269–76.

Schou, M., Weinstein. (1980). Problems of lithium maintenance treatment during pregnancy, delivery and lactation. *Agressologie*; 21(a):7–9.

Scott, D. (1992). Early identification of maternal depression as a strategy in the prevention of child abuse. *Child Abuse and Neglect*; 16:345–58.

Segraves, R. T. (1980). Marriage and mental health. *Journal of Sex and Marital Therapy*; 6 (3):187–98.

Shiono, P. H., Mills, J. L. (1984). Oral clefts and diazepam use during pregnancy (letter). *New England Journal of Medicine*; 311:919–20.

Sitland-Marken, P. et al (1989). Pharmacologic management of acute mania in pregnancy. *Journal of Clinical Psychopharmacology*; 9 April, 20:78–87.

Slayton, R. I., Soloft, P. H. (1981). Psychotic denial of third trimester pregnancy. *Journal of Clinical Psychology*; 42:471–3.

Slone, D. et al (1977). Antenatal exposure to the phenothiazines in relation to congenital malformations, prenatal mortality, birth weight and IQ score. *American Journal of Obstetrics and Gynecology*; 128:486–8.

Sokol, R. J. (1981). Alcohol and abnormal outcomes of pregnancy. *Canadian Medical Association Journal*; 143–8.

Spielvogel, A., Wile, J. (1986). Treatment of the psychotic patient. *Psychosomatics*; 27 (7):487–92.

Steiner, M. (1990). Postpartum psychiatric disorders. *Canadian Journal of Psychiatry*; February, 35:89–95.

Steiner, M., Flemming, A., Anderson, V. (1986). A psychoneuroendocrine profile for postpartum blues. In: Dennerstein, L., Fraser, I. (eds). *Hormones and Behaviour*. Amsterdam: Excerpta Medica, 327–35.

Stern, L. (ed.) (1985). *Drug use in pregnancy*. Adis Science Press.

Stern, G., Kruckman, L. (1983). Multidisciplinary perspectives on postpartum depression. *Anthropological and Social Science Medicine*; 17 (15):1027–41.

Stewart, D. E. (1985). Possible relationship of postpartum psychiatric symptoms to childbirth education programmes. *Journal of Psychosomatic Obstetrics and Gynaecology*; (4):295–301.

Surrey, J. et al (1990). Reported history of physical and sexual abuse and severity of symptomatology in women psychiatric outpatients. *American Journal of Orthopsychiatry*; 60:412–17.

Sykes, O. A., Quarries, J., Alexander, F. W. (1976). Lithium carbonate and breastfeeding. *British Medical Journal*; 2:1299.

Tamminen, T. (1988). The impact of mother's depression on her breastfeeding attitudes and experiences. *Acta Paediatrica Scandinavia Supplement*; 344: 87–94.

Tilley, D., Goldberg, S., Friedel, R. (1982). Current knowledge of tricyclic response indicators. *Psychopharmacological Bulletin*; 18:132–5.

Tong, L., Oates, K., McDowell, M. (1978). Personality development following sexual abuse. *Child Abuse and Neglect*; 11:371–83.

Tonge, B. (1986). Postnatal mood statistics. Antecedents, features and consequences. In: Dennerstein, L., Fraser, I. (eds). *Hormones and Behaviour*. Amsterdam: Excerpta Medica.

Tonge, B. J. (1984). Postnatal Mood State, Mother–Child Interaction and Child Development. Doctoral Thesis, University of Melbourne.

Trethowan, W. H., Conlon, M. P. (1965). The couvade syndrome. *British Journal of Psychiatry*; 111:57–66.

Tunnessen, W. W., Hertz, C. G. (1972). Toxic effects of lithium in newborn infants: a commentary. *Journal of Paediatrics*; 81:804–7.

Tylden, E., Dawkins, J., Colley, N. (1986). Pregnancy and opiate addiction (letter). *British Medical Journal*; 295:551–2.

Uddenberg, N. (1974). Reproduction adaption in mother and daughter. A study of personality development and adaption to motherhood. *Acta Psychiatrica Scandinavia Supplement*; 254.

Uddenberg, N., Englesson, I. (1978). Prognosis of postpartum mental disturbance: a prospective study of postpartum women and their 4½ year old children. *Acta Psychiatrica Scandinavia*; 58:201–12.

Verloove-Vanhack, S. P., Van Zeben-Van Der Aa, T. M., Verwey, R. A. (1988). Addicted mothers and premature babies: a disastrous outcome (letter). *Lancet*; 20 February: 421–2.

Visser, A. et al (1994). Psychosocial aspects of in vitro fertilization. *Journal of Psychosomatic Obstetrics and Gynaecology*; 15:35–43.

Waldby, C. (1984). The legacy of incest: short and long term effects. In: *Breaking the Silence*; 41–6.

Waring, E. M. et al (1983). Marital intimacy and mood states in a nonclinical sample. *Journal of Psychiatry*; 11:263–73.

Warner, R. H., Rossett, H. L. (1975). The effects of drinking on offspring. An historical survey of the American and British literature. *Journal of Studies on Alcohol*; 36:1395–420.

Watson, J. P. et al (1984). Psychiatric disorders in pregnancy and the first postnatal year. *British Journal of Psychiatry*; 144:453–62.

Weick, A. et al (1991). Increased sensitivity to dopaminergic stimulation precedes recurrence of affective psychosis after childbirth. Proceedings, Conference Maudsley Hospital.

Weiner, L. et al (1983). Alcohol consumption in pregnant women. *Obstetrics and Gynaecology*; 61:6–12.

Weissman, M. M. et al (1984). Psychopathology in the children (6–18 years) of depressed and normal parents. *Journal of the American Academy of Child Psychiatry*; (23):78–84.

Wheeler, B., Walton, E. (1987). Personality disturbances of adult incest victims. *Social Casework: The Journal of Contemporary Social Work*; 597–602.

Wiles, D. H, Orr, M. W., Kolakowska, T. (1978). Chlorpromazine levels in plasma and milk of nursing mothers. *British Journal of Clinical Pharmacology*; 5:272–3.

Williamen, N. E. (1989). Breastfeeding trends and patterns. *International Journal of Gynaecology and Obstetrics Supplement*; (1):145–52.

Wilson, G. S. et al (1979). The development of preschool children of heroin-addicted mothers: a controlled study. *Pediatrics*; 63:135–41.

Wilson, J. T. et al (1980). Drug excretion in human breastmilk: principles, pharmacokinetics and projected consequences. *Clinical Pharmacokinetics*; 5:1–66.

Winnicott, D. W. (1956). Primary maternal preoccupation. In: Sutherland, J. D. (ed.). *Through Pediatrics to Psychoanalysis*. The International Psycho-Analytical Library. London: Hogarth, 300–5.

Wolkind, S., Zajicek, C. E., Ghodsian, M. (1980). Continuities in maternal depression. *International Journal of Psychiatry*; 167–82.

Wrate, R. M., Roony, A. C., Thomas, P. F. (1985). Postnatal depression and child development. *British Journal of Psychiatry*; 146:622–7.

Yalom, I. D. et al (1968). Postpartum blues syndrome: a description and related variables. *Archives of General Psychiatry*; 16–27.

Zelson, C., Rubio, E., Wassenman, E. (1971). Neonatal narcotic addiction: 10 year observation. *Pediatrics*; 48:178–89.

Index

This index is arranged alphabetically word for word; **bold** entries have the fullest information; *italic* entries refer to case examples.